TAKING THE MASK OFF...

My Journey from Dr. Seuss to The Bible

KEITH L. COOPER

Author's Tranquility Press
ATLANTA, GEORGIA

Copyright © 2023 by KEITH L. COOPER

All rights reserved. No part of this publication may be reproduced, distributed or transmitted in any form or by any means, including photocopying, recording, or other electronic or mechanical methods, without the prior written permission of the publisher, except in the case of brief quotations embodied in critical reviews and certain other noncommercial uses permitted by copyright law. For permission requests, write to the publisher, addressed "Attention: Permissions Coordinator," at the address below.

KEITH L. COOPER/Author's Tranquility Press
3800 Camp Creek Pkwy SW Bldg. 1400-116 #1255
Atlanta, GA 30331, USA
www.authorstranquilitypress.com

Ordering Information:
Quantity sales. Special discounts are available on quantity purchases by corporations, associations, and others. For details, contact the "Special Sales Department" at the address above.

TAKING THE MASK OFF...: MY JOURNEY FROM DR. SEUSS TO THE BIBLE/KEITH L. COOPER
Hardback: 978-1-962859-26-4
Paperback: 978-1-960675-01-9
eBook: 978-1-960675-02-6

"...Cooper addresses the reader directly, stating plainly that this book is for people who want their lives to change. He imbues his writing with a sense of urgency—it is not enough to better yourself; you have to do it now. Italicized bullets ask scathing, pointed questions, demanding to know the obstacles in front of your happiness and pushing you to realize that there aren't any. Those who are not put off by the intensity will thrive in it, finding inspiration in Cooper's ruminations and the philosophical conclusions he draws. ..."

"Keith L. Cooper's emotionally honest memoir, TAKING THE MASK OFF (My Journey from Dr. Seuss to the Bible), offers thoughtful advice in a conversational tone."

IndieReader review
IR Rating: 4 stars (out of 5)

Contents

Acknowledgments iv
Preface vi
Introduction xiii
   My Journey From Dr. Seuss To The Bible xiii

Chapter 1 1
   Lessons From The Cabin 1
   The World Needs Responsible Parents 3
   The Long Road Home 5
   Dads Are So Smart 9
   Alaska Is Where I Belong 11
   Home Is Where You Are 13
   Sawubona 16
   Do You Play Golf? 18
   Friendship 101 21
   Where The Hell Is This Place? 26
   Gratitude At Ten Years Old 28
   Being Still Is Not Doing Nothing 33
   It's Two Thousand Feet 36
   Sometimes We Need To Follow The Shore 38
   Let's Change The Directive 41
   Green, Green Grass Of Home 45
   To The Stepparents 47
   Thank You, Mrs. Mell! 51
   Touched By An Angel Once Again 56
   It's Just Magical 61

Chapter 2 64
   My Dr. Seuss Moments—What Really Matters 64
   Round Peg, Square Hole 67
   Why Is It? 69
   Oh, Did You See That? The Horse Backed Up! 71
   The Ingredients Of The Road 74

My Transition 75
Chasing What Matters 77
Strategy Hell, Turn On The Bilge Pump 78
The Devil Made Me Do It 84
The Four Answers 87
Fly the Plane 90
I'm Under The Cloud That Looks Like A Duck 93
Put The Damn Phone Down 96
Is It Best To Be An Owl Or A Sled Dog? 100
The Revolving Door 103
Mind To Heart 105

Chapter 3 107
Nature 107
We Are All Just Snowflakes 110
The Berthoud Pass Lesson Of Life 112
Watching Nature Rest 115
The Smudge 116
The Importance Of The Deck 118
Different Views 120
I Observe 122
Shedding The Mask Of Comparison 123
What Is Our Destiny? 125
Present, No Longer Just Passing Through 127
Raton Pass: The Gateway To America's Past 129
What Does Silence Sound Like? 130
Twelve Minutes On A Path To My Purpose 131
The Foreplay Of Fog 132
The Darkness Of Anger Overcome By
The Light Of God 134
The Penetrating Glow Of Sunrise 137

Chapter 4 139
Moving Toward God, Learning To Love Myself 139
Our Daughters 141
My Son 143
The Greatest Person My Kids Never Knew 145
Pre-Combat Checks Aren't Just For Combat 148
The PAVE Matrix 154

The Great Al Jarreau 157
Threes to Fours 159
The Exit Glacier–Man, Did I Bitch 161
Faith: It's Off Or On–There's No In-Between 165
My Date With Sadie 167
The I-Should-Haves... 172
What Counts Is Getting Back Up 174
Why I Do It... 176
Four Bags Of Concrete 178
Whose Name Would I Call?.. 181

About The Author **183**

Acknowledgments

I owe so many people for my success in life that there is no way to capture even a few on this page.

I recall attending a farewell ceremony as a young lieutenant in the first unit I joined. I'll never forget the professionalism I learned from the departing leader who was being honored and his wife as they acknowledged all the wonderful support they received from all those they'd been around for the past three years. When the officer, a Vietnam veteran, spoke, he didn't talk about any of his ribbons that went from his chest to his shoulder, he didn't talk about his three tours in Vietnam, he talked about us, the young leaders enlisted and the officers in the audience. He spoke of the importance of helping one another, and ended by looking into the eyes of his lovely wife, telling her how much he loved her and then looking at us in the audience and welcoming us to his family. That's when I knew I had chosen the right occupation of service to our nation as an infantryman. I acknowledge this wonderful leader who inspired me and the many members of all ranks in our armed forces that I had the honor to serve with throughout my many years of service.

I acknowledge my therapist who encouraged me to write this memoir and provides wonderful thoughts of consideration as she continues to work with me.

I acknowledge my kids and so appreciate their love,

along with my friends who continue to inspire me.

Most of all, I acknowledge my parents, two wonderful individuals from the Greatest Generation, the WWII generation, no longer on our Earth, who made me understand so many things, who taught me so many lessons about life.

Perhaps the greatest lesson came from my father, an African American Merchant Marine Officer who went to Naval Officer Candidate School in 1943. He endured severe racism yet never said anything negative about our country or his service: a trait he learned from his father, a dentist in the Army Reserves in 1919. My dad taught me to have hope and helped me to understand how great this country is; he instilled in me things that others hear in speeches, and he taught me that failure is not when you fall, failure is when you don't get back up. I was so fortunate to have him and others from his generation in my life.

Preface

"You want me to do what?"

"I want you to write a letter to your dad telling him how you are doing, what are your regrets, what do you seek his forgiveness for, and then I want you to bring it to me," she said.

"You're kidding, right?" I replied.

"Nope, I'm expecting it in two weeks," she said firmly.

Let me back up a bit. My therapist and I have a wonderful relationship. She is a 100% wonder and tells me I'm "full of it." Hence, we are a wonderful team.

About eight years ago, as I sat in her office, my emotional index was a 3.5 out of 10. I was in the dumps. Like most situations, when it rains, it pours. I was going through a divorce, a change of jobs, and some health issues. We had a great discussion until the topic of my dad came up. It was then I shared with her how disappointed I knew he would be with me if he was alive today, given my behavior and what I'd become. I shared how I'd wanted to be like him all my life—a humble individual who never sought any corporate objectives, who treated everyone the same.

Yes, my dad is deceased, and at the time of her request to write him a letter, he had been in heaven for nineteen years, which explains the point in the opening exchange above. As we went through my many issues, her homework assignment for me was to write a letter to my dad, telling him what I'm doing and how I'm feeling, and to bring it to her. I did just that.

I found some time in my new 500 sq. ft. unfurnished studio apartment, using an unpacked box as a table, and wrote a handwritten letter to my dad, telling him what had been going on in my life. I talked about my great kids, my job, the weather, my mom in Georgia, and more. It was a great letter, full of all the positive things in my life. Why would I want to trouble my dad with bad news? He's in heaven, so the last thing he wants to hear about is complaining, right?

Well, a week later, I pulled the letter out of the box and rewrote it, this time focusing on the task my therapist initially gave me. I wrote how I felt going through a divorce, how I felt I was a failure and had let him down, how all I ever wanted was to be like him, and how, ultimately, I was ashamed of myself. It still included the positive aspects of my kids and how great they were doing, but it also included the fact that they were not speaking to me due to the divorce. It was a heartfelt, honest letter penned until late in the evening.

About three days later, I took the letter in and gave it to my therapist. She read it, handed it back, and said, "Great. Now read it to me."

I got about halfway through the letter when tears came to my eyes. I couldn't finish it. She looked at me and asked, "Why are you so hard on yourself?"

"I just don't ever want to let my dad down. I failed

PREFACE

him and I feel so bad about it."

"I don't agree with you, Keith. Before you see me again, I want you to go home and sit down, and I want you to assume your dad read your letter, and I want you to pen his response back to you."

Well, this was a real WTF moment. She was quickly losing her "wonder" with me. I said, "You want me to put myself in my dad's shoes after reading what I wrote to him and write a letter back to myself?"

"You got it. See you in two weeks," she replied.

I was in shock.

I had learned to fly a plane at fifteen and soloed it on my sixteenth birthday. I was licensed to fly a float plane at seventeen years old. I went to West Point a month after graduating from high school, and at twenty-two I had completed Army Airborne and Ranger Training.

Throughout my military career, I have jumped out of helicopters, jets, and propeller planes and spent the night outside at twenty below with no external heat source. I was serving inside the Pentagon on 9/11 when the plane hit, and then two years later I was serving in Iraq during OIF II. I've flown numerous general aviation airplanes, later becoming certified as a FAA-licensed Airline Transport Pilot. I've experienced five engine failures over the course of forty years, including three in a plane with one engine. Of all those traumatic experiences, of all the lost sleep, heartache, sadness, and frightful moments, both personally and professionally, assuming the role of my dad for this homework assignment was the absolute scariest feeling I'd ever had.

For two weeks I wrote, rewrote, cried, lost my appetite, lost weight, isolated myself, etc. Finally, the night before my next appointment with my therapist, I finished the letter.

As I drove into her office complex, I thought about reading it to her. How could I get through it this time without breaking down? Would she think it was truthful?

After arriving and sitting down, I just stared at the wall next to her chair. She asked, "How was it?"

"It was literally the hardest thing I've ever had to do in my life"

"Good."

I handed her the letter; she read it carefully, then handed it back to me. I asked if she wanted me to read it aloud like the last letter, but she said no.

I then said, "Do you think my dad would approve of the letter?"

She said calmly, "Well, if he didn't, you wouldn't have written it." She then explained that sometimes the exercise is really the event. The shedding of weight, lost appetite, and sleepless nights were my therapy to rid myself of the doubt I'd once had.

I'm sharing this experience with my therapist because, for years, I did what most do. I held it in. For eight years, I sucked it up because I'm a man, and remember, a real man shows no emotion, right? Wrong!

I recall my time during Army Ranger training in Dahlonega, GA, when, in the mountain phase, while learning the Australian rappel, it was raining, and I slipped on the cliff and banged myself up a bit. The Ranger Instructor at the top of the cliff looked down at me as I turned upside down, getting tangled in the ropes. He could see I was holding my arm and yelled, "Ranger, hurry up and get off my cliff! Remember, pain is just weakness leaving the body!"

I did as he said. I held my pain in, and for years, every time I was in pain, especially emotional, I led myself to believe it was weakness leaving and I would be stronger afterwords. My lack of understanding of what he really meant by those words, my immaturity, my stubbornness put an imprint on my life that was more confining than any mask.

It wasn't until I was watching *Saturday Night Live* (SNL) on November 7, 2020, that I snapped. I was reawakened. Ironically, it took a comedy, an SNL monologue, to recall that letter that I wrote my dad. The SNL host was talking about the mask we all wear, how we need to be more understanding and forgiving regardless of our political affiliation. In a sixteen-minute monologue, he was addressing the ills of a nation that had just gone through a horrible divisive period and needed someone to bring us together.

But I felt as if he was talking to me. It was the same feeling you experience in church when you've had a bad week and you cringe because you think the pastor is speaking directly to you. The SNL host reminded me of what I'd asked my dad for years ago in the letter I wrote. I wanted to be who he taught me to be, without any masks. I was crying because the many masks I had been wearing all those years were so evident.

- The mask of conformity in a world that so needs a change.
- The mask of happiness when I was so sad.
- The mask of success when I had fallen.
- The mask of what's important when I confused it with what's urgent.

The monologue was a mirror that brought out the problems in America and closer to home, the problems in me. I had to change my Lazy-Susan-self, showing only the parts I wanted others to see while wearing a mask that hid the parts I was ashamed of.

I decided to capture the next eighteen months of this roller coaster world and my life using the backdrop of what I learned as a kid reading Dr. Seuss at our cabin and as an adult confined during the COVID lockdown—lessons to love myself again. Yes, this was going to be another explanation to my dad, but this time it wouldn't be a letter. It would be a book. A memoir loaded completely with vulnerability and an admission of guilt, grounded in the truth. A book not only asking for forgiveness but a book that would let my dad know that even when I went down the wrong path, I really did know the right way based on his teachings to me fifty years ago.

PREFACE

At times, I fell backward to move forward.

Reading this memoir will be a journey of independent stories, from the lessons within Dr. Seuss to what I learned from my dad during our time at the cabin, to nature, and then to God. A journey from Dr. Seuss to the Bible. It is my hope that my sharing will result in your success. I hope we learn from one another. I look forward to hearing from you on my website, www.longlakelore.com. I recommend you don't try to read the entire book in one sitting. Instead, try reading story by story, taking a pause to think, and maybe discussing if a partner is nearby. As you read, try to replace my characters with those in your life.

Each story has two parts: 1) the writing itself, and 2) a few thought-provoking questions in bullet form and italicized. All writing, albeit not in any sequence, revolves around one of the four masks I was wearing and how life changed when I took them off.

Thank you for reading my book. It's now time to begin our journey. Together, let's follow the ideas in this book through your personal experience and better ourselves and those we love.

Dr. Seuss says, "Be who you are and say what you feel because those who mind don't matter and those who matter don't mind." Or, as the Bible says in Romans 12:2, "Be not conformed to this world: but be ye transformed by the renewing of your mind."

Introduction

My Journey From Dr. Seuss To The Bible

As mentioned in the preface, I finally realized just how many masks I needed to shed. To start this painful task of shedding, I relied on lessons I learned. These were lessons I learned watching cartoons, lessons from my youth growing up in the outdoors of Alaska, and lessons from watching nature. However, the most important lesson I re-learned was the greatness felt when you learn to love yourself again and focus on God. This is how my journey took me from Dr. Seuss to the Bible.

My journey was not easy; I initially put a barrier around my heart to hold in negative emotions and feelings. My first writings were all joyous, positive, and somewhat emotionless. It was during the third or fourth writing that I realized my words were coming from my mind and not my heart. At that point I began the longest journey of my life—I had to make the seemingly impossible eighteen-inch trek to move my writings from my brain to my heart. It was now time to take my many masks off, masks that felt like they were affixed to me with super glue. I knew pulling them off would undoubtedly leave open wounds. But open wounds need fresh air to heal, and I knew that sharing these writings with you would be the fresh air I needed. Yes, in the end I will have some scar tissue, but scar tissue is a small price to pay for the freedom

INTRODUCTION

of not wearing masks.

My journey led me to read many books from military leaders to religious and spiritual figures. I finally realized what others had told me all my life: God never changed; I had to be the one to change. So, I changed. Once I concluded that my issue was a problem others shared, I decided to dedicate this book to my wonderful kids as a snapshot of their dad and others who were like me.

I decided, as I wrote, that I wanted to challenge myself and invite people into my life. How would I be vulnerable? How could I improve my health? I wanted the reader to put themselves inside my heart, not my mind. Given that COVID was my pseudo-heart attack that cleared my arteries, what could I do to ensure my readers chances were minimized so they did not follow my lead?

For once, I no longer worried about disagreement. For once, I no longer wanted to be like everyone else. The blue shirts and dark blazers of the corporate world no longer fit my image. Now, it's a thermal long-sleeve t-shirt and gray pants with Timberland boots, and not to mention I'm twenty pounds lighter, work out an hour each day, and sleep eight hours each night. I was so worried about answering the question, "Is your glass half empty or half full?" and learned to rephrase it with the answer, "I'm just thankful to have a glass." I had to learn it's better to be disliked for who I am than to be loved for who I am not. This is my time to speak out. For those of you who think this book is about mental health, well, for you it might be, but for me, it's about total health.

Now you can see why I wrote this and how going back to the basics of what I learned at the cabin and what you learned from your mentors will bring us back as a nation. This book will explore why community is more important than the individual and why each of us should strive to say yes at every opportunity.

For those of you who think you are fine and I'm the one who has problems, let me run a few things by you:

- Inflation is at a forty-year high; on average, you are paying $445 per month more this year for the same things you bought last year.
- Many stocks have declined to a point many thinking about retiring within the year are now having second thoughts.
- Want to buy a house? Well, plan on paying about $824 per month more for a $500K home.
- Our climate issues are causing second order effects resulting in numerous environmental disasters.
- Our drug problem, especially with opioids and fentanyl poisoning, is out of control.
- We are among a population that will spend $320 for an oil change but won't spend $300 to see a mental health professional as part of their routine yearly exam.
- Our nation lost one million loved ones due to

- COVID, many of whom we said goodbye to through a window or on an iPad.
- We have a tyrant attempting to take over another country in Europe.
- Our country is more racially divided than ever.
- We can no longer find workers for service-related employment.
- The transportation industry is a mess. We average three railcar derailments per day and over five runway incursions per day. If that doesn't scare you, I'm not sure what will.
- The State of the Global Workplace 2022 report showed 60% of people were emotionally detached at work, with 33% feeling engaged. In the US, 50% of workers reported feeling stressed, with 41% being worried, 22% sad, and 18% angry. So, given my background as an infantry soldier, that means one in every five people you work with is angry, two out of three are emotionally detached, and every other person you meet is stressed. Unless you, as a leader, address these concerns while continuing to show yourself as an empathetic person, well, good luck keeping a steady, productive workforce.

So, given all I've written above, if you are still okay, then great; there is not much you will gain from this book. However, if some (or all) of what I have written above bothers you and you are on the path to reading this book, let's begin by putting our personal judgment of each other where it belongs: in the trash can. Just looking at the information above is enough to make anyone's head spin. So, in my mind, it's not that you or anyone else is crazy; it's that we are pretty normal people living in a crazy world. Going back to basics, asking yourself some simple questions, and reading about where I screwed up just might help you. I'm opening up to you in the hope that you can open up to others, so you can love yourself, so that you can see someone in discontent and help them to improve. No, I'm not the perfect-looking exercise instructor who opens up before every exercise to motivate you by saying, "Forget all the misery, forget all the pain, give me thirty minutes, and we are going to kill it today." I'm flawed, I'm not perfect, and I don't want you to forget the misery. I want you to remember it and, after reading this book, have a better understanding of how you can avoid it. I also want more than thirty minutes of your time. I know it's damn hard to forget anything; however, what we can do is forgive, beginning with forgiving ourselves.

Reading this book will be a journey. It is not a book you can read completely through, and it follows no particular sequence of dates. It's written for you to read a story, put the book on your lap, close your eyes, and think. It should be referenced and highlighted. I hope that you will tab and curl the pages. It should bring out some pain, pain that ultimately will pass through your strong heart, like the wind through a tattered flag, still standing and stronger. So, let's take this opportunity to

INTRODUCTION

challenge each other and open up. Let's mix it up and challenge normality, using a collection of stories from nature to civil rights to this mystery I call my wake-up call. In the end, it's my hope that you decide to journal your journey and then share it.

It's now time to begin our journey together.

Keith Cooper
Winter Park, Colorado

Chapter 1

Lessons From The Cabin

This portion of the book recounts stories from my childhood to current world events, each with a common theme of the lessons I learned from my dad while at our cabin at Long Lake, Alaska.

Each summer weekend, my dad and I would go to our cabin, our place of solace. What started as an 8' x 26' used trailer in 1968 on a piece of lakefront land later evolved into a small 24' x 28' structure built in 1972 by my dad and his friend, Jack Carl. There was no running water, hence no showers, no electricity, no TV. We had an outhouse which served us well until it rained, because the roof sometimes leaked. We washed our hands in a bucket filled with lake water and a bar of Zest set up on a tree stump. We showered by jumping into the lake, usually a warm sixty-something degrees. Entertainment was a loud AM radio placed on our kitchen table so we could listen to the Anchorage Glacier Pilots semiprofessional baseball team on Friday evenings and football games, highlighted by the Washington Huskies quarterback Sonny Sixkiller and later, Warren Moon, on Saturdays. It was the place that, as a little boy, I learned that the

CHAPTER 1

most important things are not actually "things" at all.

The mornings were highlighted with watching Dad make a pot of Folgers coffee on our gas range. There was a magic to this old coffee pot. First, water was added to the pot, then the metal strainer with coffee and stem were placed inside the pot and set on the range. Soon the bubbling coffee was visible through the little clear cap on top, then it got a bit darker, and suddenly Dad would reach over and turn the gas range off and put the coffee pot on our cast iron wood stove to keep it warm. Simultaneously, while the coffee percolated, Dad would put a slab of Hormel Black Label bacon on the skillet. Yes, a complete slab! He had that magic touch to know just when to pull the individual slices apart and put them on the plate so that they remained nice and soft. He would then cook the eggs, using the same bacon grease (Yeah, I know, very unhealthy. Truthfully, I don't think the words trans-fat, and peanut or olive oil were around back then, so we'll let this one slide.) With the bacon done, the eggs coming out of the skillet speckled with black bits of bacon grease, it was time to grab two slices of soft white bread, sit at our 4' x 2' table on our hard vinyl seats, and enjoy breakfast.

How I miss those days, and how I miss my dad. To say time heals all wounds may be true, but time also makes me understand how great my dad was and how great our time at our cabin was.

Now, let's all take a trip to my cabin!

The World Needs Responsible Parents

I miss my dad. I really miss my dad. I missed him long before he died. I missed him since I left home for West Point at the age of seventeen.

As I look up my driveway during the COVID lockdown, I see some families walking along the many trails and some along the gravel roads.

I see young kids running ahead and falling, only to have a big creature of a father come pick them up and say keep going. It's a life I'm so glad to finally see that exemplifies memories that last forever and don't cost a thing. No one will ever remember their mom's big stock bonus, but they will absolutely remember Mom and Dad walking together along the trail at 2:30 p.m. during COVID lockdown in April 2020.

I think back to the times with my dad when I see those families. The walk my dad and I did when I was eight years old, from the highway at mile marker 66 to our first plot of land on Long Lake. The trips to Wasilla, then to Cottonwood Lake, when Dad was pulling the 12′ Smoker Craft boat upstream with me inside. Or on Dad's fiftieth birthday, when he got up on two water skis and I got up on one water ski.

I remember the joy on his face when I told him I was going to West Point, and the tears we shed when friends of our family died.

I know my dad is in heaven, but his death twenty-four years ago still seems like yesterday.

CHAPTER 1

I know he's looking down on me even though I cannot see him. I know he misses me, too.

With all that I have accumulated, all that I have done, all those I have helped, I would give it all up for just five minutes of being that little boy once again on the road with my dad.

So please, moms and dads, spend time with your kids. Shed that mask of urgency to really understand what's important. Don't be in such a hurry to accumulate wealth that it sacrifices time with your kids. Be a parent, take your time to let your sons grow up to be men and your daughters grow up to be women. Trust me, you will have plenty of time when they are out of the house to accumulate wealth and material things, only to later find out how little those things really matter and ultimately how hard they are to get rid of once you have them.

- *Consider a loved one, whether they be a niece, nephew, son, or daughter. What are you going to do in your life to change so you can have more time with them?*
- *How many achievement award ceremonies, field trips, soccer games, or baseball games have you missed? Why?*

The Long Road Home

Ansel Adams, the famous twentieth-century photographer, is a favorite of mine. While I love great art and have friends who display their wonderful paintings valued in the thousands of dollars along the hallways of their beautiful homes, I proudly do the same in my hallway with my Ansel Adams prints, which cost at most a hundred dollars each including the frame. Adams, known for his photographs of the Tetons in Wyoming and spectacular photographs in New Mexico, could bring extraordinary things out of an ordinary picture.

One of my favorite Ansel Adams prints is a picture taken of a forest during the autumn. The forest is speckled with a mixture of birch and evergreen trees, with the birch trees having bright gold, orange, red, and maroon leaves. Within the forest is an old country road or trail covered by leaves that show a rain had just fallen, for the leaves have perfect circles of clear water with enough weight in the center to cause their ends to curl up.

As your eyes follow the wet leaves in the print, it's soon very clear, those wet leaves define a road with a bend. What's around the bend is left up to your imagination.

It reminds me of the scenery I would see when Dad and I headed to our cabin in Alaska, the road we would travel down every summer weekend.

CHAPTER 1

We would drive down Highway 1 to Palmer and then take Highway 3 to Willow. After turning off Highway 3, we would drive to mile marker 66, turn left into what looked like a gravel pit, and then enter what today would be labeled a trail. No respectable individual would ever drive a car down this road, but we did, every single summer weekend. I think it was the look of the single-lane muddy road that turned people off, which is probably why we rarely had any visitors.

We would then drive past the Jones' residence, which is where we would always launch our boat, because their slipway was not as steep as ours and we could back in our rear-wheel-drive 1966 Buick Wildcat with the boat on top and hopefully not get stuck. We would then drive by the Smiths', then turn into the driveway we shared with the Martins.

I marvel because back then we didn't need a map; we knew where we were, where we were going, and usually how long it would take us to get there, unless, of course, we got stuck. Now those of you who are my age remember those days; there were no cell phones, no AAA to call if you got a flat, no GPS, and you know what? We did okay, didn't we?

Once we got to the cabin, we both had our chores. I would grab a bucket, go down to the lake, and fill the bucket with water to wash our hands. Dad would prepare hot dogs in one pot and a mixture of beans and corn in another. He would call the mixture of beans and corn "succotash." Prior to it getting too dark, we would light the kerosene lantern, eat dinner, talk, and then hit the sack for the evening.

In contrast, today we have technology that not only tells us where we are but where we should be. We have let technology guide our lives instead of using technology to our benefit.

If you can't tell by now, my message is not really about vehicle capability as much as our direction in life. I can sympathize because since leaving Alaska as a teenager, I have gotten stuck on that road with all the conveniences. It seemed like the more technology out there equated to the more distractors I followed. Sometimes I put the wrong coordinates in my GPS, sometimes I didn't pay attention while my GPS was recalculating. I knew the road home, but I chose not to follow it because of what I perceived as necessities like money, security, upward progression, and all at the expense of what really matters.

In another way, I was hiding behind that mask of conformity. Since leaving the cabin, I've gotten stuck on roads our 1966 Buick Wildcat, with its rear-wheel drive and its own set of Arizona pinstripes (scratches from the brush along the road), navigated so effortlessly fifty years ago. This hurt me mentally and physically, so much so that it took its toll on relationships, and as early as twenty-eight, I began taking acid reflux medication. So, take it from someone who listened to his GPS instead of his heart. I know what I'm talking about. I'm now back on the path to follow the long road home, not necessarily to Alaska, but the road that leads me back to the

CHAPTER 1

fundamentals that made me who I am today, not who I think others want me to be. I am now like the salmon that, through instinct, is headed back up the same stream where I was born, not letting logs or bears get in my way in hopes of one day finding ultimate peace and fulfilling a legacy of making a difference.

You know, I was never as happy in my life as when I was with my dad on that narrow, muddy, and slippery road to our cabin each weekend. Although I always asked what's for dinner, I always knew what we'd have: hot dogs and succotash. Unfortunately for me, it took me fifty-plus years to realize we were never really going to our cabin—we were always headed on the long road home. What I wouldn't give for just another meal of hot dogs, white bread, succotash, and a 7Up with Dad.

- *Put the book on your lap and think. Where is your long road home?*
- *Think about your parents, your older relatives. How did they navigate pre-GPS? Did they all use AAA trip tickets, or did they instinctively have a well-known path? Why can't you now start to do the same?*
- *Tell me about a loved one in your life like my dad.*
- *What is your succotash story?*

Dads Are So Smart

"I don't want to go to the lake; I want to stay home. There's nothing to do up there. It's boring. All we do is chop wood, fish, water ski, play horseshoes, drive the boat, and hunt." These are words from an immature twelve-year-old who, in his mind, had every right to complain. That boy was me, forty-eight years ago.

Fast forward. It's 4:36 a.m., and the sun is out and the trees are casting a perfect shadow on the lake as I look out from my home in Alaska. I slept soundly for over seven hours and I'm awake sitting in my mom's recliner on June 30, 2021. The trees are still, and all I can see from either of the 5′ x 5′ windows or through any one of the other twelve windows is the lake. It glistens through the trees, saying peekaboo with each leaf that gets in the way. It is completely silent. What does the silence I'm talking about sound like? Well, picture yourself getting a hearing test and they just put you in this sound chamber. The technician puts headphones on you, and suddenly, before the first tone comes across, you hear nothing. Well, that's what it's like here.

Okay, sometimes I hear the leaves, or the lone loon on the lake bellowing a tune, or the chirping of a chipmunk, but for the most part I hear nothing. Complete silence.

As I leave the corporate world, the world that defined me by my climb up the ladder, a world that held me by a leash, a world that I mistakenly put on a mask of conformity versus change, I'm astounded at what I

CHAPTER 1

missed. The internet, social media, the 24-hour news networks have combined their efforts to turn me away from who I really am.

My dad bought our land in 1968 and built our cabin in 1972. He was never confined to anything. The only ladder he worried about was the one he used to clean the top of the windows.

Dad, you were not just smart, you were brilliant. Thank you for being my dad, and thank you for taking me to the cabin, overriding all of my teenage complaints.

- *About twenty years ago, a commercial was aired that featured celebrities drinking milk, showing their white milk mustache with the caption, "Got Milk?" Well, for those of you with kids, "Got teenagers?" You know what I'm talking about. Heck, think of yourself years ago. What brilliance did your older loved ones teach you when you were twelve to fifteen?*
- *Better yet, how are you showing your elders that you understand the lessons they taught you?*

Alaska Is Where I Belong

I decided to come home to Alaska—the state I was raised in, the state that fed me, the state that educated me, the state I always talk about. It's where the only mask I had to wear was for freezing weather while snowmobiling. None of my four masks have a role here. Alaska is a state where you are who you are, and those who mind, well, they really do not matter.

What caused this sudden decision to come back home? Well, sometimes it takes leaving Alaska, as I have, to realize what a dream it really is to live here. Being able to enjoy peace and quiet while just breathing clean air is something all of us hope for. But unfortunately, usually it's not until one or more of these benefits are denied that they're missed and greatly appreciated. I am guilty of taking Alaska for granted, similar to my prayers when I sometimes forget to thank God for the regular stuff, you know, the commodity items like waking up and breathing.

When I was in the military, during our informal time of comradery, every service member always had a place they called home. Some would tell stories of their relatives who were farmers and their desire to return home to help on their family farm after their enlistment was up. Others would talk about taking over the family construction business, being a pilot, or going back to teach and coach the high school sports team. Those places my fellow soldiers would call home were in proud small towns; some were larger ones, and

CHAPTER 1

some were even in other countries.

It was not until we served in Alaska that the question of home changed for many from where they were originally from to Alaska. For the first time, I heard my fellow soldiers respond when asked where they would like to go after retiring or serving out their enlistment with the statement, "I think I would like to just come back here. I want Alaska to be my new home, my new start."

Alaska became who they were, too, and the feeling is contagious. I'm so proud that my real home is Alaska, and I'm equally proud that so many fellow soldiers I served with chose to join me here.

- *Take a second and think as you stare out your window or into your fireplace. What state or place best defines you?*

- *When are you going to go there and plant your roots?*

Home Is Where You Are

I once wrote a story in my journal about my trip across Long Lake to see what was on the other side of the lake. The piece focused on how, for years, I had been enamored with looking across Long Lake, thinking how lucky others must be over there on the other side of the lake. Over there on the other side, the early morning sun shines through their windows. Their land looks open, with nice homes; everything seems to always be better over there.

When I finally made that trek across the lake, got out of my 9' rowboat, and stepped on the shore of "over there," I immediately turned around to look at the place I left, my cabin. I was awestruck and almost cried. I saw the solitude, the distinctiveness of the trees, the three hills from the shore to the cabin, and a piece of the trail I climbed and descended each day. I saw my dad waving to me from our deck, which he built around the trees so as not to disturb the scenery. Looking up, I saw the sun like a piercing laser shining above our roof. It seemed like part of the sun was resting near the chimney, and from the chimney I saw the smoke from the wood stove. I could not wait to get back in my boat and go back across the lake to my home, the cabin.

This lesson learned over fifty years ago taught me that life is where you are, and although for ten minutes I was "over there," I wanted to be back at my cabin. "Over there" had the sunrise; my cabin had the sunset. "Over there" had banks that were not so steep, but my

CHAPTER 1

cabin had seclusion, privacy, and trees.

Fast forward to the present day. One evening, my neighbor gave me a tour of the lake in his boat. It had been twenty-plus years since I'd been around the lake in its entirety, so this was a special treat.

What I immediately noticed upon our tour was how much things had changed. So many more homes were on the lake—probably a hundred or more—some as close as a subdivision in the city. Some homes were huge, others were small. As we traveled north, the homes got closer and closer. I saw grass greener than an Augusta golf course, and even a lawn sprinkler was going. Clearly, these were not the kinds of places I remember when I was growing up on Long Lake.

As we rounded the lake on its northern edge, the areas I thought were a swamp were now populated with homes; some even had canals through the swamp like a New Orleans bayou. We passed two homes that had nice floatplanes parked—clearly my new best friends.

We continued our trip south to see the area I lived in from the viewpoint of the lake. I could not see my cabin. As I looked at my land from the lake, I could see the different docks, but something mysterious occurred to me about my side of the lake. Truly, little had changed. I suddenly had no desire to clear my trees, plant grass, or have my home side-by-side with others. I value my privacy now more than ever.

Just like the trip I took across the lake fifty years

ago, I was once again reassured that my "over there" was here, at my cabin. My excitement about taking this boat trip had reaffirmed one thing: the more things change, the more they really stay the same. There is a saying, "You get what you get, and you don't throw a fit." I so wish I had heard that sixty years ago, as my "over there" caused me to take so many detours in life, many filled with failure.

- *What will it take for you to realize that what you have is what you need?*

- *How often have you taken a trip around your neighborhood, only to realize how wonderful the home you have really is?*

- *Everyone has an "over there" story, even in a relationship. What is yours?*

Sawubona

What floor? Hey, do you get off here? A metal box suspended by a cable that goes straight up and down, dropping us on our floor at work.

What floor? Ah, third floor: procurement; fifth floor: marketing... thanks. Then silence, because the person in the back leaning against the elevator wall was not paying any attention; they were thinking about the email they received walking from the parking garage.

For years, our jobs brought us to the same metal box. Those of higher authority had suites on the top floor with wonderful scenery; some even had a corner office.

For years, I was one of those people, checking my email from the parking lot, struggling to go higher and higher while hoping to be the last one dropped from this metal box. I was using my mask to climb a false ladder of success.

I often looked in awe at the diversity, quietness, and solitude of ten people in a metal box. Some made a million dollars a year, and some barely got by. Some were just diagnosed with cancer, and some had just learned they were pregnant. Yet, with all those feelings, they all looked the same, staring at the lights going across the top, waiting to say a polite "excuse me" prior to working their way to the elevator door to get off.

I wonder how, as humans, we will historically define elevators as a place in our lives. What will happen when we return to the new normal? Will we treasure the elevator's capability as a transport? Will we now look each other in the eye when we meet in the new post-COVID working team, or will we go back to where we were before, quiet, all facing forward, staring at the same lights indicating the floors?

There is a Zulu greeting, "Sawubona." It means, "I see you; you are important to me, and I value you."

Wouldn't it be great, as elevators are again part of our lives, if we could just say "Sawubona" to one another? Or if we'd prefer, simply "good morning" or "hello"? For those of you who find a greeting in the elevator a bit hard to do, well, maybe you should take the stairs.

My dad never had an elevator at his place of employment, just a set of wooden stairs going to his office on the second floor of a warehouse, an office he shared with four others. He always spoke to everyone and treated everyone with respect. He was the vice president of a large sporting goods company and wore gray pants and a short-sleeve shirt every day, even in the winter. If we ever got on an elevator going somewhere, he was sure to speak to everyone in a polite fashion. I still have so much to learn from him.

- *Close your eyes and think: Are you letting a metal box define your place in life?*
- *How do you let your associates and friends know they are important to you and that you value them?*

Do You Play Golf?

It was 8:45 a.m., and my son, Chris, was visiting me in Winter Park right before COVID struck. It was a somewhat weird time because COVID had been declared a pandemic, yet everything was still open. It was February 2020, and we were in for a change no one could have predicted. Earlier in the year, I had been looking at some new properties and was excited to share the news with Chris. Although I loved my home, I thought it would be cool to live on a golf course. Several of my friends lived on a golf course, and they loved it. So, my intent was to sell my home and buy a home of a similar size on the golf course across the highway, about two to three miles away. I had gone as far as picking up some brochures and taking several drives to view the perimeter of available properties, and my network of friends in real estate had assured me that selling my home would be a breeze.

I had just finished making breakfast, as Chris and I had a busy day ahead. He sat across from me, ferociously eating his bacon, eggs, and toast. What you need to understand about Chris is that he's one of those kids who stands 6'2" and weighs about 160 lbs., and nothing he eats ever fills him up. Get the picture? That morning, he was eating in a modified European style: no, not with utensils in both hands, but with food in one hand and more food in the other.

As he took a bite of bacon followed by a bite of toast,

I said, "Hey, Chris, I'm thinking about moving."

Without looking up, he replied, "Hmmm."

I then said, "I love this house, but I think I'd like to be across the highway and live on the golf course. Heck, if there was a way to move this house, I would, but I'll probably just buy a house of a similar size."

Chris looked up, a little bit of egg hanging off the right corner of his mouth, still chewing his food, and stared at me so we were eye to eye, only to say, "Do you play golf?"

It was then that I realized it wasn't Chris; it was my dad telling me to be practical. Dad always said, "Just because you can do something doesn't mean it always makes sense to do it."

What Dad was telling me, through Chris, was to be who I am and treasure it. I didn't play golf, and I wasn't planning to start playing golf, so why the hell did I want to live on a golf course? My other friends who lived on a golf course played golf, which made perfect sense.

I didn't mention moving again to Chris during his visit or since we had that exchange. The common sense he'd shown outweighed my eagerness to get what I didn't need. This wasn't a case of the grass being greener on the other side; this was a case of why do you need grass at all? That morning, there were two of us at the breakfast table; however, this time, my son was clearly the adult. He caused me to take off my mask of conformity and replace it with common sense.

CHAPTER 1

- *Take a second and think about a time when you wanted to do something that you liked the sound of but really had no business doing. How did things turn out?*
- *What lessons can you take away from "Do You Play Golf" that enable you to be more grounded?*
- *What was the most recent lesson a youngster taught you that aligned exactly with what your parents would have said?*

Friendship 101

When I was growing up, my parents had a lot of different friends. Mom had Idella, Barbara, Laverne, and Nell. Dad had Burt, Leroy, George, Freddy, Jesse, Diegel, and Harold.

Most of Dad's friends were from where he worked and were white. Most of Mom's friends were Black. Remember, Alaska's Black population in the 1960s was less than five percent of the state's population.

Regardless of race, we loved all the friends that my parents had. I marveled at my dad when he had his friends over; they played the piano, drank, and watched Dad play boogie-woogie on the piano. Mom's friends went to our tiny kitchen and just chatted. During the occasional time we had both sets of friends over, I would sit in the background and listen, learning the history of my parents as they told it to others. I felt like we were all sitting around a fire with elders, passing knowledge. I loved listening to Mr. Freddy; he owned a janitorial service in town and had the best stories. Every time he came over, he told the same stories; the only difference depended on the amount of alcohol he had drank before telling the story. Freddy could not get through any story without laughing, especially the stories about the fish that got away, so it was always a challenge to figure out if Mom and Dad were laughing at Freddy's story or laughing at Freddy as he laughed. What amazing times!

Since those times fifty years ago, I have owned and

CHAPTER 1

lived in many homes, each at least four to five times the size of the home I grew up in, yet none of them had nearly the amount of love and laughter my parents' house did. I long to have the relationships with my friends that my parents had with theirs. It is probably for that reason that in both of my homes now, I have a no-media room: the living room, where nothing but music, board games, talk, yoga, and laughter are allowed; no cell phones, TV, etc. We do something unique in the Cooper household called talk, and do you know what? Once it starts, no one even looks for their phone. As a side note, to date, at sixty-two years old, I've yet to be defeated at a game of Twister by anyone; something about the call, right foot blue or left hand red, always causes my opponent to fall!

Of all the friends my dad had, two stand out: Harold Mason and his wife, Lee, or otherwise known to me as Mr. Harold and Mrs. Lee. I was taught to show every adult respect. Every adult was addressed as a Mr. or Mrs. with the first or last name, period. Truthfully, it baffles me today when I see a five-year-old calling a fifty-year-old by their first name. Now, am I judging? Of course, I am, and the truth is that I won't change because respect is nonnegotiable in my book.

Like many, Mr. Harold and Mrs. Lee came to Alaska in the late sixties looking for work. My dad hired both of them: Mr. Harold as a truck driver and Mrs. Lee as an administrative clerk in the front office. Almost immediately, Mr. Harold and my dad hit it off as friends. My dad normally maintained some distance with those he worked with, but he let Mr. Harold in much closer than normal. They would both go with Dad and me to the cabin almost every summer weekend.

About fifty percent of the time, I would talk Mrs. Lee into making some of those great pancakes. She used a mix from Krusteaz, a seasoned cast iron skillet, and bacon grease; yes, it's truly something. With a cigarette in her mouth, coffee percolating, grease spattering all over, and the baseball game playing loudly in the background on the AM radio, this was breakfast at its best. The pancakes all came out light and fluffy, with a semi-hard crust on the edge. I could eat a hundred of them. Those pancakes, combined with my dad's bacon and Mr. Harold's toast, made for some of the best breakfasts I have ever had. Having breakfast with Mrs. Lee and Mr. Harold was something to look forward to each time they came up.

Unfortunately, in 1972, at the age of 45, Mr. Harold died of a massive heart attack in his sleep. I remember the night like it was yesterday. My parents and I were talking at the kitchen table when Mrs. Lee called, saying they'd rushed Mr. Harold to the hospital. We only had rotary phones at the time, so when the phone rang late, it was usually bad news. My mom answered the phone, then passed it to my dad to talk. Both looked a bit flushed. My mom told me to go to bed, and they left for the hospital, saying Mr. Harold was sick.

The next thing I remember was hearing a noise in the kitchen. I got out of bed in my white briefs and walked into the kitchen, where I saw my parents and Mrs. Lee

CHAPTER 1

sitting around our kitchen table, crying.

My dad looked up and said, "Son, we lost Mr. Harold today," and he gave me a hug. I then gave Mrs. Lee a hug, went back to my room, and cried. We lost a part of ourselves that night; we lost a key member of our family.

I often recall the great times we had with Mrs. Lee and Mr. Harold now, and a smile comes to my face way before a tear comes to my eye. The friendship my dad had, the happiness I saw on his face—I never had to ask what made Mr. Harold so special given all the friends my dad had. Simply put, it was Mr. Harold's sincerity; none of us ever had to wear a mask of any sort. My dad and Mr. Harold loved each other like brothers; they defended one another, cared for one another, and respected one another. During a time of such racial divide in our nation, you would never know without seeing them that my dad was Black and Mr. Harold was white. This was Alaska, and friendship among different races was not uncommon. When I think of real friendship today, my models are Mr. Harold and my dad.

Both are in heaven now, enjoying their endless friendship, talking about the big one that got away, and loving one another. My sincere hope as they look down on Earth and see me, my kids, my friends, and my happiness is that they both will agree they are responsible for my understanding of what a friend really is.

About fifteen years ago, there was a TV commercial about a young lady who moved back home to live with her parents because she felt they were lonely. It was a car commercial, highlighting the versatility of a new four-wheel-drive.

The commercial opens with mom and dad, in their late fifties or early sixties, leaving the house in the evening on a date. They get into their SUV, go to a restaurant, have a wonderful time, and return home to find their daughter, late twenties to early thirties, sitting at the table alone on Facebook, bragging about how many new friends she has.

The commercial cuts to the next day, to a similar scene, except this time the parents leave mid-afternoon and go surfing with another couple. The daughter, sitting at the table alone on her computer, looks up after they leave and says, "I feel so sorry for them; they don't have any friends."

I think you can see where this is going. Whether you are on Facebook or another app is not the issue. Having friends you can count on is. My recommendation: don't count your Facebook friends as friends; count your friends who don't require you to wear a mask, as your friends.

- *How do you define a friend versus an acquaintance?*
- *How do you allow your young kids to address elders?*
- *Who were the friends you remember your parents loving the most? How does the friendship you have with your closest friends today compare to that friendship your parents had with their friends?*

Where The Hell Is This Place?

It's fifty-four degrees outside. It's a blistering sixty degrees inside. The rain is hitting the lake, making the surface look like a smooth fabric with clear polka dots. The buzz of mosquitoes in the distance is drowned out by the crackling of burning wood in the fireplace. The sink and toilet work fine, but there is no hot water. I tried to Google the nearest plumber, but there is no internet service. I then tried to call a friend to come help me, but the phones don't work here. So, I turned on the TV, only to see static because there was no TV either.

I thought, "Where the hell is this place?"

I thought about taking a walk outside, but where would I go? There are no walking paths, and there are no forest rangers with gray shirts and green pants handing out brochures. There is only the outdoors. Okay, last time, "Where the hell are you? Why are you here? Why don't you leave?" The answer to all those questions is "I am home. I am at Long Lake."

This comment caused me to understand that the conveniences of home apply most when you are away from home, very similar to the masks we wear when we are out of our comfort zone. Because whether it be a favorite lake, river, place in a city park, or somewhere outside, you feel at home. When you are home, conveniences really do not matter, and masks are not needed.

- *Take a second and think: When was the last time you were in a place with little or no conveniences? What was going on in your mind when you were there?*

Gratitude At Ten Years Old

When I was a young boy growing up in Alaska, we were fortunate to have snowmobiles. We used them to get in and out of our cabin during the few times we went in the winter and sometimes just to have fun on the local lakes around Anchorage, primarily Sand Lake or Mirror Lake. I used to love going to Sand Lake during the winter because it was close by, and they also had ice car races, which were really nothing more than race cars with spikes on the tires. It was cool to sit on my snowmobile and watch the cars slip and slide; some would even hit the snowbank! It was winter, it was Alaska, and this was entertainment.

One weekend, my dad and I left early on a Saturday morning to go up to our cabin for the night. My mom had prepared macaroni and cheese casserole, along with some leftover meatloaf she wrapped in foil, so we could simply heat up our meal on our wood stove and not be bothered with cooking. Keep in mind that the temperature was often twenty to forty degrees below zero, so taking three hours to heat our cabin, followed by cooking a regular meal, would have meant we were not able to eat until very late at night.

As we neared our turnoff from the highway, we pulled our car over onto a side road, unloaded our snowmobiles off the trailer, and decided to save time traveling to our cabin by cutting across the lake versus following the much longer road.

As we loaded our equipment onto the toboggan that

would carry our supplies, we looked down the road at the lake. It was a pristine morning. There was fresh snow with no tracks, and it was unseasonably warm, around twenty degrees above zero, still below freezing. What a great day, or so we thought. My dad tied the rope of the toboggan carrying our supplies to his snowmobile; he would lead, and I would follow in case anything fell off. As we entered the lake, I noticed my dad was going slower than normal. Then suddenly, so was I. We were stuck.

What we did not know was that the lake was experiencing a condition called overflow. Overflow usually occurs when, after the lake is frozen solid and several snowfalls blanket it, there is a warming trend, usually caused by the hot sun beating down on the snow, which causes the snow to partially melt into a slush. Then, several days later, it gets colder, and it snows on top of the slush. So, overflow is like a body of water that structurally resembles a key lime pie. The pie crust is the solid ice, the lime filling is the slush that got us stuck, and the sweet topping is the snow that covers the slush. Unfortunately, unless you can look directly down on a body of water by flying over it, overflow is difficult to see.

Overflow can be a killer—not because you might fall through the ice, but because once you get stuck in the middle of a lake and become wet, you are setting yourself up for hypothermia, which, if left untreated, can lead to death. There are cases every year of snowmobiles being caught in the overflow, and people have to build a fire once back on land to dry out before they go any further because they are soaking wet, and the temperatures, once the short daylight falls into night, can easily reach below zero.

So, after we got each other unstuck, we proceeded across the lake about two hundred yards before I got stuck again. After the third time holding us up, my dad knew we would not make it to our cabin before dark. Alaska in the winter at that latitude has, at most, four hours of daylight each day. Going back was also a nonstarter because the trail we used was obviously slush-filled, so we took a sharp turn east toward the shore and stopped at the first cabin to spend the night.

We found the uninhabited cabin locked, which was not unexpected. My dad quickly broke the lock and started the log fire inside. This was to be our home for the night. Toward the evening, Dad put the leftovers Mom had made, still wrapped in foil, on the wood stove. We grabbed some utensils from the owners' cabin and ate our food right from the foil. Macaroni has never tasted so good.

The next morning was clear, still dark, and very cold. My dad knew this was our best chance to depart back across the frozen lake, for the cold temperatures during the night made our previous trail of slush now hard ice, our escape route for a short trip back to the car. So, at about 7 a.m., we loaded up all our equipment on the toboggan, closed the door, and followed the trail we got stuck on yesterday back to the car without incident. We loaded our snowmobiles up, and we were home before noon.

I recall my mom being pretty surprised that we got

home so early because we had never gotten home that early before. I quickly told Mom the story, and she laughed, not really understanding what we had gone through.

The next day, my dad called Willow Hardware to try to locate the property owner and let them know what we did and why we did it. He wanted to reimburse the owner for the loss and damage to the lock. This was a time before cell phones, in 1970, and the local hardware store was the focal point where everyone knew what was going on. Even if the hardware store didn't have the number, they knew someone who knew someone, so it was only a matter of time before you got a call back.

About a week later, after calling the hardware store to leave a message for the owner, Dad got a call from the owner of the cabin we broke into. Not only did the owner of the cabin, Mr. Hatcher, understand why we broke in, he refused to take any money for the damage to the lock. He said we did the right thing, and he would have done the same thing himself.

From that day on, the next time we went to our cabin, we always left our door unlocked. At ten years old, I had learned the importance of helping one another, that kindness is not weakness, and of gratitude, something I give my dad and Mr. Hatcher credit for.

Unfortunately for me, after departing Long Lake as a teenager and moving into adulthood, my actions did not reflect that story. Based on my personal experiences of being taken advantage of by others who were primarily focused on themselves, I tended to trust people less and

CHAPTER 1

less. I formed a callus and put aside gratitude while focusing on the mask of conformity. I have now gone back to revisit the lesson I learned from Mr. Hatcher and my dad fifty years ago, and I'm working on trusting and relying on people more.

- *When was the last time you gave someone a second chance? Tell me your gratitude story.*
- *What spiritual doors have you unlocked in your life to allow those who care about you to get closer?*

Being Still Is Not Doing Nothing

I was fortunate to read a book by Father Rohr titled *Falling Upward*. Reading this fantastic book reminded me of the Lay's potato chip commercial that aired about thirty years ago—the one where they challenge everyone to just eat one. The commercial has a gospel choir in the background in a courtroom, and after the accused fails to eat just one and starts munching on a second and third chip, the jury stands up and sings, "He tried, but he couldn't do it; he tried, but he couldn't do it; no one can eat just one."

Well, reading Father Rohr is like eating Lay's potato chips; you just can't stop once you start.

Father Rohr's book focuses on the second part of our lives, hence the term "falling forward." He challenges us to really define how we are going to make a difference. For many who are still trying to climb the first half of their lives, so focused on everyday events that they are not even thinking about tomorrow, the book is a real eye-opener.

At the end of the book, Father Rohr summarizes things very well. He puts pseudo-metrics in place for people like me when one enters the second half of life. One statement he makes is fascinating. It simply says, "Be still, be still."[1]

In our everyday rush to multitask, Zoom, care for our families, perform well at our jobs, achieve that to-

---

[1] Father Rohr, *Falling Upward* (San Francisco, Jossey-Bass, 2011), p. 162.

do list, go-go, or talk-talk if we can't go, I find my most valuable time each day is when I wake up, walk downstairs, and just sit in complete silence, staring out the window. Not moving, just thinking, just being still, whether it is daylight or darkness.

It is when I am in the trance of being still that my problems go away, my mind is cleansed, and I'm ready to take on the challenge of the day. I do not think about my to-do list or my not-to-do list. I have no phone or iPad; my lights are off; nothing is on. Even my Apple Watch, which periodically tells me to breathe throughout the day, is sitting upstairs, charging on my desk.

I remember my time at the cabin some fifty years ago, when I would see my dad just sitting in his favorite hard vinyl chair, looking out at the lake. Whether I was reading a comic book or building a model plane, Dad could just sit. Often, I would ask him, "How can you just sit there?", to which he would just smile and say, "One day you will understand." Well, now, after fifty years, I understand.

Being still is not doing nothing. Being still means allowing your heart to lead. It is not reminiscing; it is more like not trying to remember. It is putting aside the mask of what is urgent and focusing on what is important. If you could recreate that feeling you have every night before falling asleep in bed while sitting wide awake, well, that is being still.

This transition has been tough, sometimes frustrating, but completely worth it. I now love being still, and I love Father Rohr for opening my mind.

- *When was the last time you did absolutely nothing? Was it really nothing, or were you being still?*
- *What is on your to-do list today?*
- *More importantly, what can you take off your to-do list now that you have read this? How will this change your approach to tomorrow?*
- *Try doing nothing tomorrow for ten minutes. You will find those ten minutes will soon grow to twenty, then thirty.*
- *Ahh, I get it, you have kids, the dog needs your attention, your boss sends an email at 6 a.m. Well, wake up earlier. Trust me, once you get ten minutes of freedom to do nothing, you will find another ten minutes by cutting out the unnecessary things in your life. By the way, when your boss sends an email at 6 a.m., you shouldn't be near your phone; and if you are, don't answer it! Just because they don't have a life doesn't mean you shouldn't have one.*

It's Two Thousand Feet

Growing up, I always wanted to be a pilot like my dad. Not an airline pilot but a bush pilot, or maybe a Marine or Navy fighter pilot, like Alaska's former governor Jay Hammond.

I recall looking out the kitchen window many times at the Chugach Mountains, often to see only a layer of clouds blanketing the mountaintops and rain. I would then remark to my dad, "How can those small planes fly when the clouds are so low?"

I remember him saying, "As long as you can see midway up the mountain, you have two thousand feet—plenty of altitude to fly safely."

Today, I am fortunate to live near the mountains at my home in Winter Park, Colorado.

As I look out my windows at the Continental Divide, I have a picturesque view of the many ski runs. Sometimes, as the clouds hover over the ski run and nearby Shadow Mountain, I think back to the optimism of my dad, who has been in heaven for over twenty-six years, a dad who I miss so much every day, and I say out loud, "Hey Dad, it looks like two thousand feet."

To which he would say, "Hey, big guy, go ski."

And I do.

- *In Colorado, we have a saying: There is never any bad weather, just bad clothes. Who are you going to tell during times of misery, fog, and division:*

"Hey, it's two thousand feet, let's go"?

- How can we use the attitude of "it's 2000 feet, let's go" to make our nation better?

Sometimes We Need To Follow The Shore

When I was sixteen, I received my Student Pilot certificate in a small, two-seat Cessna 150. Per the regulations for a student pilot, I could fly alone in a predefined area in weather conditions approved by my instructor, or I could fly with an instructor. I could not fly with anyone else in the plane, I could not take passengers, and I could not go further than twenty-five miles without having an instructor sign off on each trip. Taking passengers required a private pilot license, and you had to be seventeen years old to take the test for a private license. So, I had an entire year to do a lot of flying alone. To build hours of experience, I would get my instructor's permission to take numerous solo cross-country trips.

One day after getting the required permission, I departed Anchorage and headed south across Turnagain Arm toward the town of Homer, about a hundred and fifty miles away. After landing and walking around the many planes at the airport, I took off and headed north toward Kenai. Normally, I would follow the coastal road past Anchor Point, always keeping the road below me as a safe place to land.

However, as I proceeded from Homer toward a town called Soldotna, I started following my pencil mark on the map rather than my instincts. Before I knew it, I was near the shore of Tustumena Lake, a vast lake probably twenty-five to thirty miles long and five to ten miles wide, and from the altitude I was flying at, it looked like an ocean: all I could see was water, and my plane had one engine and three small wheels. Spoiler alert: planes on wheels don't float.

I knew, based on my straight line on the map, that I would cross the lake and only travel six miles over water. But that was six miles in a single-engine plane flying at an altitude that provided a gliding distance of one and a half miles should the engine quit, with water at about fifty degrees Fahrenheit. At this point, had I been smarter than scared, I would have asked, "Can I swim the remaining mile and a half should my engine quit halfway across the lake?" But no, I kept plugging ahead toward the shore of what looked like the Pacific Ocean. No wonder sixteen-year-olds cannot vote or buy liquor.

As I crossed the shoreline, I looked at my compass heading, rechecked my azimuth, and rechecked my map, only to find that the water had no definable landmarks. Once I was over the shore surrounded by water, it seemed as if the air became more turbulent, and the engine started sounding a bit rough. The truth was that the turbulence did not increase, and the engine was fine, but I was getting a bit scared, and my conscience took over. I quickly turned left and just followed the shoreline of the lake, probably adding another ten to twenty minutes to my flight to Soldotna.

I never told anyone what happened because, really, nothing happened except that a young kid learned a very important lesson. Sometimes we need to stray from the

CHAPTER 1

lines we draw. Planning, including drawing the lines, is important, but sometimes the best way between points is not a straight line; sometimes each of us needs to take the time to follow the shore.

I wish I did not follow all the straight lines of my life or the steps of a ladder leaning against the wrong wall. I wish I had disengaged my brain more often and realized that constantly following straight lines may only take you to the wrong place a bit faster.

- *Is life a straight line for you, or do you tend to follow the shore?*
- *Tell me about a time you took the back roads instead of the interstate. Wasn't it breathtaking? Maybe those back roads are now your shore.*

Let's Change The Directive

When I was a teenager, I used to watch *Leave It to Beaver*. During one episode, Beaver and his brother, Wally, were helping their dad build a bomb shelter in the backyard. Remember, the show was cast in the sixties, during the height of the Cold War between the US and the Soviet Union. This was a time when sirens would sound at noon every Wednesday so that students at school could practice hiding under their desks and those in the street could move to bomb shelters in case a nuclear war between the Soviet Union and the US occurred.

As the show played on, the sons, the dad, and a big machine with its operator were in the backyard, digging this hole to put the bomb shelter in. During one of the breaks for refreshments, Beaver asked his dad who they were planning to invite inside their bomb shelter should a national emergency really happen. The dad replied, "Well, just our family."

Then the son starts rattling off the names of his friends he wanted to invite because he could not imagine being without them. Shortly thereafter, Beaver's brother, Wally, comes out and asks the same question about his friends, including the mischievous Eddie Haskel. To which the dad interrupts and says, "Kids, this is for us, for our family."

The next day, the man operating the machinery and the dad were in the backyard, both wondering where the kids were. Out of the blue came both kids, only to

CHAPTER 1

say, "Dad, can we talk?" The dad put down his shovel and walked over to the picnic table where the kids were, and they said, "Dad, I know this is important, and you paid a lot of money to save our lives, but if something happens and all our friends die and we live, what's there to live for?"[2]

I did not think about that scene from *Leave It to Beaver* until fifty years later, when President Obama took office and all the violent, racial, and hateful rhetoric that was always present became even more prevalent. People of all beliefs were buying bug-out bags filled with medical supplies and food just in case a civil war broke out. In some cases, bug-out bags make perfect sense, like during hurricanes, floods, and snowstorms that could isolate someone for days without power.

But if we experience a large nuclear explosion, a pandemic, or a civil war in which everyone is affected and the end is in sight, what is there to live for if our loved ones are lost? Why are we here? I think it does not matter who was elected—Trump, Bush, Obama, or Biden. If our nation is so fragile that because of an election we are going to have a civil war and kill one another, then what is there to live for?

My dad was a quiet man who never discussed hate; he never discussed the racism I know he faced during his time in the Navy during WWII. He only discussed love and getting along. Not only did he discuss it, he practiced it. Knowing that, it became clear to me that the dad in the series *Leave It to Beaver* was focused on

---

[2] *Leave It to Beaver*, Joe Connelly (producer), 1957–1963, CBS.

putting a bomb shelter in because of the seemingly urgent prospect of nuclear war, but he forgot that what's important, family and friends, surpass that urgency.

Now, my personal pledge is not to prepare for a disastrous outcome but to shape the environment through respect and love, so the chances of a disastrous outcome are reduced.

I recall a famous ESPN sports anchor, Stuart Scott, who had fought cancer for years. Two weeks before he died, a physically weak Stuart Scott gave a speech at the ESPY Awards. During his speech, Stuart said, "When you die it does not mean that you lose to cancer. You beat cancer for how you live, why you live, and in the manner which you live, not how you die."[3]

As we navigate through and beyond COVID, let's understand that, as a society, we will be judged for how we lived and how we prevented future disasters, not how we ran from them. Let us change the directive so we can work together to respect and celebrate our differences without reverting to fighting and building bomb shelters.

- *What are you doing to ensure we don't turn our world over to our kids worse than our parents turned it over to us? What, if anything, needs to change in your life?*

---

[3] Stuart Scott, ESPY Award Speech, July 16th, 2014.

CHAPTER 1

- *What can we do to refocus our thoughts toward building shelters for those in need so they can be part of our community, versus bomb shelters for those who want to avoid a community?*

Green, Green Grass Of Home

The year is 1968, and it's hard to tell if my mom's love for the iconic Welsh entertainer Tom Jones is greater than her love for my dad. If there was one show she watched every week, it was the *This Is Tom Jones* show, and if any of us kids talked during the show, we were skinned!

Tom Jones was the real deal. Simply put, the world stopped whatever they were doing to watch the *This Is Tom Jones* show. Even my dad watched, although I think his rationale was looking more at the women in the audience who took off their bras to throw at Tom than listening to him sing.

There was one song that Tom Jones sang, though never on his show, but its meaning stayed with me, as it was my dad's favorite. I remember we would have guests over at the house, and after listening to Ray Charles sing "I Can't Stop Loving You" or Redd Foxx on an album telling his jokes, things would get serious, and my dad would play a song by Tom Jones called "The Green, Green Grass of Home." It was a story of a man who left home and how he envisioned his return.

The song was a hit but never reached number one in the US, but the meaning preserved itself over time. Back in 1968, one could visualize Tom Jones talking about a Vietnam veteran returning home or a family initially separated by divorce now giving one another a second chance. I now know my dad was way ahead of

CHAPTER 1

his time, for he had a vision when he played that song—a vision of acceptance—using the backdrop of a song by a white Welshman, playing among friends of many backgrounds, singing about the return of those who left our society, all the while showing how we should welcome them back.

Today, that same song could portray an incarcerated prisoner who is returning to society after properly serving time, a soldier who served our nation and is now back in our community, or a COVID patient who recently recovered and has been discharged from the hospital. Regardless of who they might be, let's use the lesson my dad put in place years ago, putting race aside, to ensure that all of us can welcome those who have departed back to a place they can call the green, green grass of home.

- *What are you doing to keep the home fires burning in your neighborhood to give those coming back a warm welcome and a chance for success?*

To The Stepparents

I have a friend who was going through a difficult time and feeling a bit down due to not being a blood relative of another family member. She felt that since she was the stepparent, her advice would not be taken seriously by the family member she so wanted to help. She, the stepparent, had always felt as if she was an outsider.

After hearing her story, I told her, "I feel your apprehension based on the announcement of your stepdaughter's unexpected pregnancy. I appreciate you sharing."

I then explained that what I have to say is something that I used to shun, but as I have gotten older, I now want to share.

In 1959, my mom, a divorced mother of a seven-year-old girl, fell in love with a military man, my biological father, while living with him in Kansas City. Just after my birth, he got out of the military and joined the FAA. At that time, FAA radar operators were needed, so he traveled to Alaska to monitor the radar stations, which primarily tracked commercial airline traffic from Alaska to the Pacific. Keep in mind that this was pre-GPS and pre-visual omni-range, and all the planes going from the US to Asia had to stop in either Hawaii or Alaska for fuel. The planes departing Alaska would then fly the great circle route along the Aleutian Islands to Japan, the route that my biological father was assigned to track.

CHAPTER 1

After he left Kansas City to get started on his job in Alaska, my mom, sister, and I followed shortly afterward. I was still an infant, and my sister, Beatrice, was now eight years old.

Mom arrived with me and my sister in the village of Iliamna, Alaska, in 1960. For the life of me, I do not know what happened between my biological father and my mom; she never told me. But what I do know is that they broke up. So, you have a Black woman in Alaska with me and my sister in 1960. My mom then moved to Anchorage, with a population of about 44,000, to begin her new life—a life in a state that had just become a state, a life with two Black kids and no father in 1960. Although I absolutely sympathize with single women of all backgrounds raising families alone today, I can't imagine what my mom went through in 1960.

My mom made some new friends and got a job in a warehouse, while her friends took turns watching over me and my sister. At her new job, she met this great man, who just happened to be her boss, another Black man, a WWII veteran, and they fell in love. After she moved to another job, they married, and he took her, me, and my sister into his home, where we lived as a family.

That man, Felix Cooper, is my father. He is the only man I will ever acknowledge as my father. Fast forward to when I was in high school in the late seventies and selected as the senior class president, among other accolades, including selection to the incoming class at West Point, when my biological dad, who abandoned me in 1960, came back into the picture. He had not talked to me, called me, or done anything for me for seventeen years, but now he had a desire to come back into my life. He had pancreatic cancer and less than ninety days to live. He contacted my mom and expressed a desire to attend my high school graduation, where I would speak as the senior class president alongside the US Senator from Alaska, Ted Stevens, and several others. I remember looking at my mom and telling her, "I don't want him to come; I have a dad who did not abandon me." I later found out that my biological father died two weeks after I graduated. I didn't shed a tear, for he, in my mind, was not and never would be my dad.

So, like I told my friend, who was apprehensive, do not think for one second that you are not key and influential in the lives of your kids, even if they are not your biological kids. You are! I write to you as a child of the sixties who was adopted and raised by a wonderful man who I adore more than anyone in the world. To this day, twenty-six years after my dad died, I never say stepdad, and I never talk about my biological father. The man who took me in and raised me until his death when I was thirty-seven was my dad.

To all parents who are stepping up and taking responsibility, regardless of whether you are with your partner or not, be proud. Thanks to your efforts, your kids and stepchildren will grow up to be as wonderful as you are. What the world needs now is love—sweet love. My dad gave that to me in 1960 until the day he died.

CHAPTER 1

- *How many people do you know that are not blood parents but are the best real parents? Have you told them that?*
- *At the end of the day, a child needs a parent to show up, they don't care about a DNA test. So, to all parents, just be a parent!*

Thank You, Mrs. Mell!

Mrs. Mell was my Algebra II teacher in high school. She was a tough but fair teacher who taught me lessons about life beyond Math. My biggest regret is never personally thanking her for the effect her leadership had on my life.

The story began on the last day of my junior year of high school. It was report card day, and in those days, we received a piece of paper with our grade on it. Nothing was computerized or automated, nor did we have the internet. Mrs. Mell walked around to our desks, thanked us for our work, and wished us a wonderful summer. She told each of us something special she liked about us as she approached our desk, and then she handed us a piece of paper with our grade. She was a person who knew more about each one of us than our parents did, very similar to the great teachers we have today.

Well, long story short, I received a B, not an A. My grade did not come as a surprise, for all the scores I'd received made it apparent that I would get a B. However, my dad had always given me $5 for each A I received and nothing for a B or below. So, making the honor roll continuously with 4 As and 3 Bs or 6 As and a B was nice, but that magic of straight As never ever reached my report card, let alone my dad's wallet.

Alaska had a policy that high school students needed four credits of English and three credits of Math to graduate. Each year counted as a credit. So, given I'd taken both Math and English since the 9th grade, I was, in my mind, done with Math and could cruise to victory by taking Office Aide as a senior instead of pre-Calculus, thereby assuring me of that A grade I so desperately wanted to get that extra $5. (Laugh if you want, but $5 in 1976 was a lot of money. In my first job in 1974 as a high school sophomore stocking shelves in a warehouse, I made $2.10 an hour, before tax.)

So, upon the dismissal of class before heading to my locker, I stopped by Mrs. Mell's desk and thanked her, to which she replied, "See you next year."

I then smiled and told her if she did, it would be in the hallway because I was not taking Math as a senior. I went over the logic of only having to take the state-required three years of Math and reminded her that I had fulfilled my graduation requirement.

I then said, "By the way, my dad gives me $5 for each A and nothing for a B, so I'm shooting for straight As next year and not taking math because I have never made an A in Math."

Well, she smiled and said, "Okay, have a good summer."

That evening, as I was sitting at the dining room table watching TV, I heard my dad arrive at about the regular time. Mom was already home. He walked in with the paper under his arm, a bag carrying a few groceries, and a six-pack of Carling Black Label beer. He walked by, said his usual "hello" as he unloaded his arms, and then went into the bedroom to take off his shirt and come back in with his white t-shirt and slippers. He sat down in the chair behind me and opened the paper, then he started talking. He said, "A friend of yours called me today."

Now, this was the last day of school, either a Wednesday or a Thursday, and no friend of mine would have called my dad. I mean, really. So, I turned and looked at him, very puzzled, as I thought, what did I do? I then asked, "Who called you?"

He announced to both me and my mom, who happened to be in the kitchen cooking, that Mrs. Mell, my Math teacher, had called him at work. "She said she talked with you, and you had no intention of taking Math as a senior. She said you were a wonderful student, and she knew taking pre-Calculus next year as a senior would help you."

I then said, "Dad, she's right, I have no intention of taking Math. I don't have to. The state rules for graduation state only three years are needed, and I have met those requirements. Besides, Dad, you give me $5 for an A and nothing for a B, and I can tell you I'm planning on making straight As next year."

My dad popped the tab of his beer, then shuffled the newspaper to the sports section and simply said, "You're taking Math next year."

I was absolutely devastated, but I knew I would be taking Math for a fourth year. I didn't know it then, but I was developing a mask of conformity. Thank goodness my dad snatched it off my face.

The next year, I did not make straight As. I continued

CHAPTER 1

to get a B in Math, and I did not get that $5. But the pre-Calculus course helped get me into West Point. West Point enabled me to be a successful Army leader, and the Army sent me to the Colorado School of Mines, where I received a master's in math, and well, the rest is history.

Mrs. Mell, a teacher from the greatest generation, did not let grades or money deter her from making a call to my dad. I owe her so much that even as I write this, forty-seven years later, tears still come to my eyes.

So, for those of you out there chasing money or grades or performance reports at work, I want you to look back at your life and see who your Mrs. Mell was and send them a thank-you note. I don't even want to think about where I would be today had I taken the easy route of $5 and an A. Our teachers change our lives, and we should be appreciative and grateful. Each of you should consider doing what I did and writing your version of a thank you to Mrs. Mell!

- *There is a reason kids talk as positively about their teachers as their parents. Teachers know kids and the potential of kids better than most parents. Teachers do not get stock bonuses; teachers do not make the money you and I do. They have a higher calling, a calling that resonates around the success of our kids.*
- *Before you get upset because your kid came home with a grade you think was too low, just maybe, before picking up your cell phone, pick up your*

shoes and go have a respectful conversation with the teacher about your child. Should the teacher call you, listen before defending your child then ask the all-important question: What can I do as a parent to work with the teacher so my kid can become a better student?

- *Who was your Mrs. Mell in high school? Have you told them thank you?*

Touched By An Angel Once Again

One of the fondest memories I have of my dad is from 1995. At that time, he was in his early seventies and fighting late-stage lung cancer. It was when we were both at our cabin, and I was a young Army major who took the weekend off from my posting at Ft. Wainwright, Alaska, to spend time with him. God had blessed me and my family with this opportunity to be in Alaska during my dad's cancer fight. Mom and Dad were able to see our two young kids, Chris and Megan, during Dad's final two wonderful years on Earth.

The cabin had also progressed from the days of lake water and Zest soap on the tree stump. Dad had installed electricity, plumbing, and even a four-foot-tall TV antenna on top of the roof. Personally, I don't think it had anything to do with his initiative but everything to do with my mom threatening not to come to the cabin unless he got rid of the outhouse, and he'd promised her hot water for a shower.

While sitting at our fake Formica dining room table on hard plastic yellow vinyl chairs—the kind of vinyl chairs that start to peel after ten years and then cut your butt every time you sit on them—I watched the ducks and the loons as a few boats passed by, then I got up and moved five feet to the living room, where Dad sat. He watched two shows every weekend because he still worked during the weekdays. One of those shows was *In the Heat of the Night*. Dad loved Carroll O'Connor and Howard Rollins. Then he would turn to *Touched by an*

Angel with Della Reese, Roma Downey, and the Angel of Death played by John Dye.

The TV was positioned on the living room table—it was one of those TVs with a thirteen-inch screen and a thirty-inch depth. It was hooked up to a cable that went out the door and up the outside wall to an antenna on the roof. Depending on the weather, we could usually get three clear channels, sometimes even five or six. The weekly series *Touched by an Angel* came on. This series always warmed my heart, but in truth, I wasn't an avid watcher of the show. However, I loved the opening when the three cast members, all portraying angels, were shown riding in Della's big Cadillac convertible along a lonely stretch of highway, all happily singing.

In one episode, a family is gathered at their parents' home to say their final goodbyes to their father, who is bedridden and undergoing home hospice care.

The episode opens with the usual family arrivals, hugs, and crying, then shows everybody visiting the upstairs bedroom where the father lies. Each visit inside the bedroom is characterized by smiles, love, and friendly chatter of the good times they shared as a family. After the siblings had time to speak alone with their father, they go downstairs to the living room. Once they are all assembled, the fighting begins.

Sound familiar? Arguments erupt, everything from how one kid never loved dad as much as the other to how one older sibling, going through a separation, can't keep her life together.

Then suddenly, the other siblings start picking on the

CHAPTER 1

youngest, saying things like, "Why are you even here? He's not even your dad." Boom, bombshell. The mother, overhearing the fighting, comes rushing in from the kitchen, yelling, "That's enough!", to which the youngest daughter replies, "Enough what? What are you talking about, Mom?"

Well, then the eldest daughter, who is going through her own personal separation, starts in with a tirade of how twenty-plus years ago, while she was in junior high school, some of her friends worked with their mom, a waitress at the time, at the restaurant across from the motel in town. Her friends were part-time busboys and busgirls. The eldest daughter tells the assembled family members how embarrassed she was at school because her friends would regularly see their mom and their dad's boss leave the restaurant and go to the motel while dad was at work.

The siblings glance at the mom, who then lowers her head, for there is truth to the story.

As everyone sits quietly staring at one another, the youngest runs upstairs, only to see Andrew, the Angel of Death, standing beside her father. Her father has just died. She tries to shake him awake, but it is too late. The youngest goes downstairs to interrupt the bickering family to tell them what has happened, and together they go upstairs to say goodbye and cry around the father. In the background, Della and Roma intermingle with the family, and when the family goes back downstairs to call an ambulance, both Della and Roma convince the Angel of Death, Andrew, to bring the dad back for just a few minutes so that he could heal his family. Andrew does just that.

After the mom calls the ambulance, the family moves from quiet mourning downstairs to more bickering about the mom's affair. It is dig after dig. Suddenly, they hear creaking from the stairs; it is the dad, with no IV, no oxygen, in just in a gown, holding the banister, walking downstairs. He doesn't come close enough for them to touch him, and when they see him, they all sit down in shock. He says, "I hear the fighting, and it needs to stop." He looks at the youngest daughter and says, "I am your father, as I am theirs. When I discovered my wife was having an affair, I approached my boss and said stop, and it stopped. Regardless of what a blood test reveals, I love each one of you the same, and I love my wife. Each of you is mine, and never forget I am your father."[4]

After the father is done speaking, Andrew comes down the stairs, gently grabs the father's arm, and they both walk through the closed door arm in arm to heaven.

I'm writing this to you on February 2, 2022, at 4:12 a.m., twenty-seven years since the show ended, twenty-six years since my dad passed, and almost two years since losing my mom, and I still cry. I was so blessed to have my dad take me as his child, unite us as a family when I was eight months old, and raise me to be the man I am today. He provided a unity so strong that he did not need to bring us together upon his death, for we already were.

---

[4] *Touched by an Angel*, John Masius (creator) and Martha Williamson (executive producer), 1994–2003, CBS.

CHAPTER 1

- *My dad, thankfully, never put a mask on. Had I continued to emulate him during my adult years, I would not be writing this book.*
- *To all of you who are raising a family in a respectful way, thank you!*

It's Just Magical

It's 4:10 a.m., and the daylight pierces the bedroom window like a laser going through a 2′ x 2′ opening. I am awake; she is not. The only sound is her constant wood cutting as she rests, which in reality is not annoying but reassuring. She has traveled over two thousand miles with me to a place she had not been before, to this new environment called Alaska.

You see, six weeks before, I'd said I would be departing for Alaska, as I always did each summer. This time, however, she interrupted and said, "I want to go."

Well, after taking several previous trips together and having a wonderful time, I figured she would enjoy Alaska, so I said, "Sure."

I know at the time she probably thought, "Yeah right, he's taking me to Alaska; sure he will." But after buying the ticket and departing less than two weeks later, I think the anxiety and excitement set in for her, for she was now really going to Alaska.

After a long journey and our arrival in a rainy Anchorage, we set off. We took a short jaunt around the city, and I showed her where I grew up. Then we were off to my cabin.

We exited Highway 3 (Alaska only has three highways, ingeniously numbered 1, 2, and 3) at Willow, and we drove along a paved road five miles from the highway until reaching a small dirt road: Long Lake Shores. I saw her eyes widen. An adventure that began

CHAPTER 1

twenty-four hours ago, with little sleep and one stop at the grocery store, had her eyes pegged on the scenery as we traveled two hundred meters along a dirt road.

We made the last turn up my private drive and proceeded up the hill under a canopy of drooping aspen trees as if we were entering the Bat Cave, all arching over a road covered with last year's leaves like an Ansel Adams poster of an autumn day in the woods. She was all eyes. The tall birch trees greeted us like we were in a receiving line driving to Wonderland. It was a cloudy day, but it didn't matter; the view was clear. We left the world of pavement for a natural paradise.

The leaves on the trees were a green that only a second grader using Crayola crayons to color a poster could hope to match, and as we crested the hill, we saw the brown aluminum roof, a brown that matched the soil, and then the entire back of the cabin. She looked through the windshield, almost coming off her seat to get a better view. She was like a kid in the zoo, putting their face close to the glass to view the animals. I looked into her eyes as she saw the cabin. They were welling up with tears.

We parked and unloaded the car, putting everything on the kitchen counter. As I put everything away, I looked through the doorway to the living room and saw her sitting quietly on the sofa, just staring. I couldn't tell if she was focused on the rain, as it looked like pin pricks on a gray blanket of water, or if it was the Norman Rockwell prints that hung on the walls. All I knew was that as she looked out, tears streamed down her face like Soap Box Derby Cars racing downhill on her cheeks. "It's magical."

I was folding the paper grocery bags. "What did you say?"

She said softly, "This place, it's just magical. The feeling you get, I can see why you and your dad loved it here."

I walked over and sat next to her as she talked about her father. How he loved the solitude, the outdoors, and places like this. As she talked, I knew his spirit was there with us. I personally think her father would have wanted her to see the cabin, the special place I call home. Although the place was not special to her father, the feeling she had was one he probably would have wanted her to have: a feeling of magic. The peace and serenity of the cabin instantly gave her the warmth, security, and happiness it's given so many others, but no one ever said it like she did. Her watery eyes peered through the five-foot windows toward the lake; she simply said, "It's magical," and well, she was right.

- *As you sit down, think about your magical place. What makes it so special? The place, the memories, or both?*
- *Have you ever taken anyone to your magical place? What was their reaction?*

Chapter 2

My Dr. Seuss Moments—What Really Matters

The next set of essays focuses on things I let get to me that I really should not have. Things I spent too much time worrying about that really did not matter to those I loved, or those who loved me. Things like promotions or fitting in, things like initial failure with a job, things like being afraid to say, "I don't know."

I recall an emotional experience a while back that caused some upheaval in my life. It was something that could have been embarrassing and traumatic, and at the time, all I could think about was my reputation and all the work I had done. It was a time in my life when I thought those who were close to me would come to my immediate aid, but the truth is that very few did.

It's astonishing to me just how quiet people you think are your close friends can be when you are going through turmoil. I felt like I had Ebola or COVID, and they were distancing themselves at a time when I really needed them. Later, when I asked some of them why they were not around, knowing what I was going through, the answer was always the same. They were giving me time and space. Of course, they were! I felt like I was a zebra in a herd of zebras on *The Discovery Channel* show, and the lion had singled me out. It felt like the rest of the zebras had made it to safety and were now looking at me, talking among one another, saying, "Man, I'm glad it's not me. Good luck with that lion, Keith; call me if you make it out of there, buddy."

Let me offer some thoughts: People going through turmoil, whether it be the death of a loved one, a departure from a job, or the loss of a relationship, don't need time. They need real friends. And for a second thought, the ones who rarely ask for help are often the ones who need it the most.

Surprisingly, in my case, those who I never expected to, those initially not so close to me, immediately reached out. People from work, most in non-executive positions as well as from other companies, sent me all kinds of correspondence, and some even offered to help. People who I didn't know outside of work now became acquaintances; people who were acquaintances became friends; and those so-called very good friends I thought I had, well, although I later forgave them, I no longer associated myself with them.

My healing began when one former female acquaintance, now a great friend, sent me a box of chewing gum in the mail. She could not come to visit, as it was the beginning of the COVID lockdown and most states had already imposed travel restrictions. The box with five Chicklet-like candies simply said, "Let that shit go." She convinced me not only to let that issue go from my mind but to let people associated with that issue go as well. Her comment was later reinforced when I was listening to a discussion while studying the Bible verse

Philippians 3:13–14, which focuses on forgetting those things that are behind. Our discussion began with one member talking about leaving material things behind. Another member further commented that it's not just about material things. He mentioned that many of us tend to make big mistakes by focusing on all those who have left our lives when, in truth, we should focus on those who remain. At that point, I knew this discussion was my real Dr. Seuss-to-the-Bible moment because those who left me no longer mattered.

"Be who you are and say what you feel because those who mind don't matter, and those who matter don't mind."

My takeaways as I went through this period were the following:

- *How important it is to forgive.*
- *I was so focused on being accepted that I stopped being who I was.*
- *If you can't see what you're looking for, see what's there.*

Round Peg, Square Hole

"You're a bit 'abby normal'; maybe you should change so we can be better together," said a woman I used to love.

"No, you don't fit in, but I hired you to stand out," said the hiring manager, who counseled me several times for not conforming.

"You're supposed to know how to play basketball, but you don't like basketball. Every Black person likes basketball; what's wrong with you?" say some acquaintances.

All my life, from being put in special education for a speech impediment during my elementary school years to being the only Black person in many of my classes to not playing sports in high school, I was different. While I appreciated the benefits and lessons of sports, I was never good at team sports. I recall being so proud of my kids when they got the high school athletic letter I never had, because at least they fit in.

Our culture is one of belonging. Fitting in is for those who rise to the top, and those who don't are set aside. A couple of weeks ago, a friend asked me if I felt successful. I said no, and she was aghast. She started rattling off my achievements, and I started rattling off my failures. We both listened in amazement. We were two people looking at success in different ways.

So, what defines our success? Do successful people fit

CHAPTER 2

in while others don't? Am I a failure for not fitting in? All my life, I have been different; I've stuck out according to others. Maybe that's why I've realized that not only will I be alone, but maybe I should be content and happy with being alone. Maybe, just maybe, my round hole is really square after all, and those who continually criticize me for not wearing the mask of conformity, well, truthfully, now they no longer matter.

- *The premise of you "should" or are "supposed to be" is based on people who conform, who have either not tried anything else or failed at what you are doing. Why would you, as great as you are, want to be part of a team, a group, or an organization that does things the same way with no input for creativity? The truth is if someone wants what was done before, why do they need you? And more importantly, why do you need them?*

- *Put the book on your lap, look straight ahead wherever you are, and just clear your mind for three seconds. Ask yourself, are you trying to fit in the wrong hole or are you reshaping the one you are in?*

- *What are you going to do to ensure that you matter, regardless of the opinions of those who may mind?*

Why Is It?

Why is it that we look at the fireplace for hours but won't look into a loved one's eyes for ten minutes?

Why is it that we tell our dogs we love them every time we see them but tell our loved ones only on special occasions?

Why is it that we will tell our friends they look good, tell our coworkers how happy we are to see them, but criticize our partner when they are five minutes late getting ready so they look good with us?

Why is it that we will make time for a subordinate to come spill their guts on any problem, from their marriage to their work, as part of our open-door policy, but when our relationship is on the rocks, we don't want to talk about it?

Why is it that we will sandwich our time with our loved ones between two immovable scheduled events rather than make time for them when we are open?

Why is it that we will spend $50,000 for a new second vehicle to pull our boat or trailer but not $12 for flowers for a loved one on the way home from the supermarket, and then wonder why we don't get laid more often?

Why is it that we will wash our cars but not the dishes?

Why is it that we serve our friends before our partners?

Why is it that we will show a happier self to others?

Why is it that we will talk at parties for hours yet ride home with our loved ones in silence?

Why is it that we will tell the truth to the court but withhold information from our loved ones?

Why is it that we will take our car in for a $297 oil change and an $82 tire rotation but won't spend one hour per quarter with a mental health professional?

Well, I don't know why, but I know I was guilty of each of these things. I know I was wrong, and I can tell you I'm damn sure going to stop doing them!

- *Are your priorities in order? If not, which ones are you going to change?*

Oh, Did You See That? The Horse Backed Up!

When I was nine, I went to see a movie with my friend, BJ, who was like an older brother to me. He was the son of my father's coworkers and best friends, Lee and Harold Mason, the Mrs. Lee and Mr. Harold from Chapter 1.

It was 1969, and BJ and I sat in the movie theater to watch the John Wayne classic *True Grit*. John Wayne portrays an old, alcoholic lawman named Rooster Cogburn who helps a little girl get revenge for her father's death. Rooster Cogburn is introduced to the stubborn little girl after she is seen going store to store along a boardwalk of shops, asking each store owner if they know where Rooster Cogburn is.

The last person the girl asks about is Mr. Cogburn, who points across the dirt road and tells her it's the man right over there with the horse.

She replies, "That old coot?"

The old man tells her she better not tell him that, but yes, he's the one backing up the horse. Immediately the camera swings over to John Wayne, who is looking over his shoulder as one would in his car and backing up a horse with supplies to a loading dock.[5]

At the time, the movie theater erupted with laughter. People broke all norms, considering the theater was

---

[5] *True Grit*, Charles Portis (writer) and Hal Wallis (producer), 1969, Paramount.

relatively silent. Everyone said, "Hey, did you see that? John Wayne was backing up the horse!" One after another, elbowing each other, it got to the point that most of us missed the entire next scene due to the noise. It was clear that seeing a horse back up caused many in the theater to lose sight of the real purpose of the plot in the movie—getting the man who killed the young girl's father. Again, it gets back to the purpose of what we set out to do.

I often think of how many times I became enamored with the "horse backing up," so to speak, the action of something occurring other than the planned result. Many of us find the cheapest airline ticket only to wind up stopping two or three times before a destination and thereby spending more money at each of the stops, not to mention cancellations, hotels, or the chance of being late due to weather or mechanical problems. Instead, we could have just paid extra for a nonstop ticket.

We often forget that the purpose of our trip is to see our loved ones, and time is money. I personally have let the "horse backing up" take my focus away from what was important, all for the purpose of conformity.

So, next time we see a horse backing up in our lives, let's grin instead of laugh and not lose sight of the rest of the picture.

- *Describe a time in your life when you let the distraction become the main event. What did you do to get back on track?*

- *Sit back and think: Are all areas of non-conformity in your life making your internal headlines? If so, why? Because those who matter really don't mind, so why should you?*

The Ingredients Of The Road

The precautions taken to abide by the many states' stay-at-home orders were immense. Without going into the details of what the outcomes of our economy were, let's all agree that suffering occurred and still occurs. Many, including myself, have lost what matters in our lives: loved ones, jobs, our health, etc. Our world has changed.

But let's step back and look at the entire mountain. What have many of us learned? Well, we've learned that love conquers all, we've learned an appreciation for one another, and we've reconnected with our beliefs.

Sometimes precautions seem like roadblocks, yet throughout our history, Americans have learned to make the roadblocks part of the road. We don't look at a crevasse as a reason not to climb a mountain; we simply put a ladder across it and keep on going. I've yet to hear someone say I need to travel from San Francisco to Oakland, but I'll need to cross the bridge first. That bridge is now just part of the road.

As we come out of COVID, let's incorporate our lessons learned as we would a bridge over an obstacle to a new and better destination.

- *What are the obstacles along your journey? Which of those obstacles can you build a bridge over? When are you going to start?*

My Transition

Father Rohr writes in his book, *Falling Upward*, "Our mature years are characterized by a bright sadness and a sober happiness."[6]

Wow, what a statement! And how true! But perhaps more telling is what he did not write, a statement that says, "Our mature years have a bright happiness."

In my mind, there is something sad about growing old. Not the aspect of approaching death, but more along the lines of the uncertainty of how much time you have remaining on Earth to make the difference you set out to make.

In light of this, my metrics have changed from achieving to believing. I am navigating from where I am, not from where I wish I was. The good part is that the foundation for wisdom, knowledge, and understanding is set. The sobering part comes into play when you are faced with how much time you have to really make that difference and focus on what matters.

To amplify this, I have begun my own word transition that describes my journey using a from-to approach:

From	To
Goal Oriented	Just Being Oriented
Achievement Based	Foundation Based
Financial Growth	Giving

---

[6] Father Rohr, *Falling Upward*, p. 117.

Check the Block to Get Ahead	Refrain from Routine
Go-Go	Sensing and Appreciating Where I Am
Family Growth	Community Love
Sex	Compassion
Things	Things That Matter
Things That Take Me Places	Enjoying the Places Those Things Take Me
Have	Give

- *What block of words above best describe your change? Why?*

Chasing What Matters

For years, I have climbed the ladders of military and corporate hierarchies under the impression that each upward rung was a symbol of success. Sometimes I slipped, sometimes I jumped a rung, but regardless, I climbed.

It was only when I was forced to let go of the rungs, or, in layman's terms, fall off the ladder, that I realized I was never climbing. I was surviving. Those rungs that I held so tightly were never holding me up; they were keeping me away. Once I fell and hit the ground, I finally realized that it was I who lacked faith to grow. I lacked faith to follow my heart, and I lacked faith in believing God would provide. I chased what could be counted rather than what mattered. I was more focused on being liked than being admired.

Now that I'm back on solid ground, I have begun to rebuild my faith, and if one day I decide to climb another ladder, the foundation of that ladder will be rooted in faith and spirituality.

- *How many times have you fallen off your ladder?*
- *If your four closest friends were asked if they liked or admired you, what would they say?*
- *What foundation are you now establishing for your ladder?*
- *Are you still climbing a ladder or is your journey more lateral like that of scaffolding?*

Strategy Hell, Turn On The Bilge Pump

One year I had the opportunity to attend a business conference with a friend of a sister company. You know, the yearly conference where the senior leadership of the company gets together to focus on events from the previous and upcoming years.

The conference began with an icebreaker the night before: a few drinks, a few hors d'oeuvres, and the most senior leaders wearing polo shirts and sport coats with their engraved name tags so you knew whom you were speaking with. It's a time of comradery where everyone is extremely friendly and all leaders make themselves available to talk with the young people and mingle with the older, established leaders. After a few drinks, most attendees moved to their rooms to finish the day's emails or just to go to sleep; very few, if any, remained until late.

The next day, after breakfast, the CEO kicked everything off and gave the opening remarks, welcoming everyone and discussing the day's agenda. He set high expectations and encouraged everyone to participate. He bent over backward to welcome new lower-level participants and ensure that everyone knew they were to be treated as equals during the conference.

Following the opening remarks, the senior vice presidents from the different divisions rotated up onto the stage for their presentations. I found one presentation, the Human Resources presentation, particularly interesting because there was a part of it that had a discussion by an outside leader on diversity. It was very telling when I looked around to see how many senior leaders had phone calls during that part and had to leave the presentation, only to be found during the next break standing by the Starbucks cart with their coffee half gone. To the credit of the CEO and CFO, however, they stayed for the diversity presentation and were super participants. I turned to my friend, who invited me, and told him how impressed I was with his senior leadership who stayed.

After three presentations and a coffee break, it was time for the pitch everyone was waiting for. Strategy. The strategy team's presentation was the last before lunch, and everyone piled in to hear how the company was planning to grow during the next five years. The finance team had already been briefed on the previous and current numbers. Now it was time to see the future, and as an outsider, I could tell the excitement was building.

Once we were seated, my friend leaned over to me and said, "Here we are about to hear from the VP of Strategy." He commented that in his last job before joining this company, the VP of Strategy was the corporate guy who hired consultants who were his old friends to put charts together that were meaningless before the ink dried.

Strategy leaders were known to blame their failed plans on poor execution by the General Managers, and after three years and changing the five-year outlook five times, they all started looking for another job. Yeah, those people.

CHAPTER 2

We shared a chuckle, only to realize later how right he was.

So, the VP of Strategy got up, walked onto the stage, and loosened his tie. He then took off his sport coat, placing it on a nearby chair. I mean, he looked like Jim Cramer on *Mad Money*. He began with the same rosy language, thanking the great leadership of the CEO and the General Managers, his team, etc. He then talked about the economy and politics, including his well-known connections to the Hill, with whom he'd spoken on the phone during the past week.

Then came slide four—yep, the infamous slide four. I will never forget slide four of the presentation because a hero emerged from the audience when the slide showed exponential future growth for the next five years. You know the slide that causes the "oohs" and "aahs" along with claps? The slide that causes even the VP of Strategy to take a step back, smile, and loosen his tie a little bit more? Yeah, that slide.

You see, slide four showed nothing but growth in a known political climate of contention. I found it a little ironic that this briefing occurred right after a new US president was elected who promised to end the war in Iraq, and well, most of the company's revenue came from selling war stuff. Regardless, the briefer was the VP of Strategy, and I was a guest.

After the "oohs" and "aahs" subsided, the VP of Strategy asked if there were any questions on the previous slides. Well, he had thoroughly briefed four slides, talked about his connections on the Hill, and mentioned how much the company was going to grow. Who could have any questions? Well, no one except one person, my friend Alex, who had invited me.

Alex, albeit somewhat new, was clearly a rising star in this company; he was not yet a VP but was on track to become one, at least before he had asked the question.

The VP called on Alex, and Alex stood up and said, "Sir, I'm Alex, a director who runs a small program. Thank you for inviting me to this forum. May I ask a question?"

The VP replied, "Of course, but please call me Dave. We don't do that sir stuff here; we are all equals on the same team."

The VPs glared at Alex like lasers drilling a hole through the side of his head. "Well, Dave," said Alex, "I spent a few years in the military prior to coming to this company."

Alex continued. "When I read the 10K report to shareholders, it echoed what the finance team just briefed; we didn't meet our financial goal last year, when we were supplying the war effort. We now have a new administration that's promised to end the Iraq War, where we got a huge percentage of our revenue from. Given the different political parties in Congress, should we face sequestration, that means no new work and only eighty percent of funding on contracts in place will occur. Sir, with all due respect, from where I sit, through no fault of yours or anyone in this room, the environment we face is one causing our trajectory to be that of a sinking ship. It seems you're trying to set an

CHAPTER 2

azimuth when we are underwater. Sir we don't need strategy; we need a bilge pump."

Thank God for Alex.

Well, that did not go over too well. But the funny thing was, after Alex sat down, the staring from the other VPs toward Alex stopped, and the CEO asked the VP of Strategy to explain. The VP, along with five of his minions, each standing up in support of their sinking boss, failed. When the strategic babble ended, the CEO turned to Alex and said, "We'll get back to you."

Fast forward: the company did not meet its numbers the next year or the year after, the CEO retired, and the VP of Strategy and his team also left. As for Alex, well, Alex didn't do any better and left the company shortly thereafter.

I often think of that story and relate it to life. I've often been on the trajectory of a sinking ship, and while gurgling underwater, I have tried to find an azimuth before hitting my internal bilge pump to breathe. I've been in relationships in which both of us felt so overwhelmed that all we needed at the time was to find our way out of being submerged. Finally, the bilge pump I turned on was therapy.

Yes, Alex was the wisest person in the room, much wiser than I was, and he lives in my heart as someone who was not afraid to tell the truth, because the truth always matters the most.

All of us, at one time or another, need to just stop and float and not be so concerned about direction. Alex gave me some advice I've used for a long time: When you are sinking, hit the bilge pump to get back on top, then worry about the direction you eventually want to go. Navigating while underwater only works for submarines, not relationships.

- *Is there an Alex in your life? Tell me about them.*
- *Tell me about a time you forgot to turn the bilge pump on, maybe in a relationship?*

The Devil Made Me Do It

The devil knows Scripture. Pastor Eric Smith of the United Methodist Church in Park Hill, a Denver suburb—the church I belonged to for five years—was known for letting us know that the devil was smart. He would often say, "It's not enough to just recite Scripture; you need to know it and believe it." Pastor Smith was also known for telling the story of a bumper sticker he saw on a car as he drove to church one day. It was someone's version of The Lord's Prayer, where the part of "Lead me not into temptation" was followed by "Don't worry, we can find it all by ourselves."

Remembering Pastor Smith leads me to recall a famous 1960s icon, Flip Wilson. Wilson, a great comedian, broke the color barrier, and during a time of severe racial issues, for an hour every week, he made everyone who watched his show laugh. Flip Wilson was the entertainer, the Tom Jones equivalent of comedy, during a very tough time in our nation's history. For two hours each week, we, all people in our divided nation transcending through civil rights, could count on *The Flip Wilson Show* and *This Is Tom Jones* to relax and laugh together.

Two skits by Flip Wilson that come to mind are "Here Comes the Judge" and "The Devil Made Me Do It."

The first skit, "Here Comes the Judge," portrayed Flip Wilson in a judge's outfit, siding with the defendants in the most ridiculous cases and letting off people who would normally be convicted. This reversal of logic, combined with Flip Wilson's swag of a walk, made all of us watching fall off our chairs laughing.

The second skit, "The Devil Made Me Do It," focused on things he did or was accused of as a mock defendant that did not look good in the eyes of the community. Flip's response when asked by the judge why he did such a bad thing was always, "The devil made me do it."

At the time, with the Vietnam War, the Civil Rights Movement, and our country's many problems, I saw comedians like Flip Wilson, Carol Burnett, and Bob Newhart and shows like *Rowan & Martin's Laugh-In* and *Sanford and Son,* without using one cuss word, break barriers and make us come to the evening table to laugh.

As we continue our education and focus on what's right when we are the judge in real life, let's also include accountability. "The Devil Made Me Do It" was a popular skit that provided comical relief in the 1960s, but the devil is present everywhere, so let's continue to laugh at the comedy aspects of what the devil made Flip Wilson do as a skit on his show, but let's all understand free will is alive and no one can make us do anything. Therefore, we must hold ourselves accountable for our own actions. Flip Wilson made me laugh for an hour each week by not conforming to accepted or expected behavior.

Unfortunately for me, I thought the lesson he taught me only applied to comedy when, in truth, it applied to life. I initially made the tragic mistake of trying to walk with God while holding hands with the devil. I should have taken my mask of conformity off much sooner, and when I did something wrong, I should have blamed

CHAPTER 2

myself and been accountable, not the devil.

- *Every comedy skit has a bit of truth, and in this case it's about accountability. Tell me how you felt when you first took accountability for your actions.*
- *What has comedy taught you about your life and the changes you need to make? Whom are you walking with?*

The Four Answers

By nature, I'm a bystander. Of the many leadership qualities, I am the one whose self-described personality takes everything in and then summarily reports out.

Given this personality trait, I tend to come across as quiet when, in fact, my brain is moving about 200 miles an hour. In social settings, I'm often taken aback by arguments, especially politics. Now, personally, I never open a political discussion with anyone unless I know them; it's just too risky. Sports, weather, the best places to live, and favorite foods are among my first choices to start a discussion. But again, as a bystander, I'm not likely to start any discussion.

I usually find myself between the group of people who know just enough to think they are right and the group that knows just enough to know they are not wrong. And as you would expect, the truth always lies somewhere in the middle, which is why I treasure being a bystander.

When I was a captain in the Army, I was assigned to the Pentagon as a staff officer. As part of our staff officer orientation, we were herded into an auditorium and listened for eight hours to a series of briefers come and go before us. They gave us pointers to help us do our jobs.

One briefing made a lasting memory. An old brigadier general from our public affairs office came to discuss the importance of not talking to the press unless

CHAPTER 2

you know what you're talking about. He made it a point to let us know that, regardless of our rank, given our access and location of work at the Pentagon, the press considers us "Army Spokespersons," and he was right.

To make his point, he put up a view graph. For those of you who are young, think pre-PowerPoint and imagine a blank sheet of acetate that you can draw on. Then picture that acetate on a projector that projects the image on the acetate to a screen. Make sense? Now think of four squares, like you used to play in elementary school. Each square had two letters. He proceeded to tell us that every subject in life falls within these four squares. You either K/K, or know what you know; DK/DK, or don't know what you don't know; K/DK, or know what you don't know; or DK/K, or don't know what you know.

He then took his pointer and hit the screen so hard that he tore a hole in the squares that had a DK/DK and a DK/K. His point was clear: We are all now Army Spokespersons, and if we are asked a question that we are not sure about, we should say, "I don't know."

As I look at our society now fighting to get answers on racism, crime, and inflation with some people thinking they are right and others knowing they are not wrong, I often think of that old general. What a lesson he could teach our politicians today! I'm still waiting for the first politician to say with sincerity, "I don't know," and for the public to appreciate that answer, because it's the truth.

The one thing I admired about my dad's generation is

that they for sure knew what they knew, and with that knowledge, they built the greatest country on Earth.

- *Take a deep breath. When was the last time you answered a question when you should have just said, "I don't know?"*
- *What will be your answer the next time when you really don't know?*
- *Are your kids/students able to tell you they don't know without fear?*

Fly the Plane

Upon my retirement from military service, I read and reread numerous books and articles on business. My intent was to gain the currency about business I had lost while in the military, so when asked the famous question by recruiters regarding any recent books I'd read, I could always answer with something relevant. The readings served me well; the different opinions of the authors presented a menu from which I could craft a unique thought on many topics.

Of all my readings, it's hard to say which one was my favorite or which one taught me the most because they all added something to my knowledge. Choosing a favorite book is like a parent deciding which kid they like best, so instead of picking favorites, let me tell you the one that taught me the biggest life lessons. And unfortunately for me, although I read it, I did not understand it. Had I followed it, I would be in a much different place in life.

Stephen Covey wrote *The Seven Habits of Highly Effective People*. In the book, he emphasizes that one should know the difference between "urgent and important."

"What is important is rarely urgent, and what is urgent is seldom important."[7] So, what's important? I thought I knew the difference. I mean, what's urgent must be important, right? Wrong. I have now

---

[7] Steven Covey, *The Seven Habits of Highly Effective People* (Los Angeles, Free Press, 1989).

developed my own personal interpretation for what's urgent and important. What's urgent is your boss's email; what's important is your family. What's urgent is answering your cell phone; what's important is listening to your kids read. What's urgent is getting up at 5:00 a.m., taking a shower, putting on your work clothes, eating burnt toast, and rushing out the door at 6:30 a.m. to sit in traffic for an hour just to make it to work by 7:30 a.m. to look at emails and drink more coffee. What's important is rolling over at 5:00 a.m., holding your partner who has a stomachache until 7:00 a.m., making coffee and breakfast for the kids, taking your coffee in the basement, then turning on your computer at 7:30 a.m., and working from home that day. Don't get me wrong; faced with a cut artery, a broken leg, and a diagnosis of cancer, you need to stop bleeding first. Just don't forget that the most important step in all those life-threatening scenarios above is to continue to live.

During pilot training, the first thing all prospective pilots are taught when faced with an emergency is to always fly the plane. It doesn't matter if the engine quits, if you're lost, or if you smell smoke; you always fly the plane. Finding your location and diagnosing the cause of the engine failure seem like common-sense first steps, but they aren't. You must first fly the plane and continue to fly the plane, or nothing else that you do will matter.

It amazes me that for someone who has survived five engine failures because I first "flew the plane," I could not apply the same logic of putting my partner first in

CHAPTER 2

relationships. For years, I confused the two, wearing the mask of urgency rather than taking it off to see what was important. Don't you do the same. Your family is the most important thing in your life; always pay attention to them first.

- *Think about what you have let migrate from being urgent to important that really isn't? What has that cost you?*

I'm Under The Cloud That Looks Like A Duck

Back in the early eighties, the Army developed three centers focused entirely on training our Army against the Soviet Union. Over the years, each of the three training centers evolved to reflect the changing threats in the world.

On the surface, the training centers were nothing but land. Each represented an automated wonderland, keeping track of every piece of equipment and engagement. One training center in California, dubbed the National Training Center, or NTC, was on a piece of land the size of Rhode Island.

During my first visit to the NTC in 1985, I was awestruck at the size and magnitude, not to mention the difficulty of navigating pre-GPS across this vast land with just a map and compass.

The truth is, navigating during an exercise was not nearly as hard as finding the After-Action Review site, which was always tucked in a crevasse on the side of a mountain, with the location only given out two hours before the review. Most of the exercises were two weeks in length and consisted of approximately ten engagements, meaning most senior leaders did not get much sleep.

One significant memory of the two-week exercise I participated in was listening to the radio chatter between the lost junior leader, a lieutenant, and a loud

CHAPTER 2

battalion executive officer (XO), a senior officer with the rank of major. The conversation went something like this.

The XO asked the junior leader, "Where are you?"

"Um, I'm getting my coordinates now; wait one," replied the junior leader.

"I don't wait one," replied the XO. "You need to tell me where you are now. I'm moving artillery into location to fire, and they cannot fire over your location."

This dialogue went on and on for what seemed to be fifteen minutes but, in reality, was about two minutes. Keep in mind that it was the desert, the temperature was over 100 degrees Fahrenheit, tempers were flaring, and everyone was sleep-deprived. The next transmission, about a minute later, came from the lost junior leader, who, clear as day, replied, "Sir, I'm under the cloud that looks like a duck."

At the time, that comment made for a lot of laughs, even in the heat, and in truth, the NTC was very well automated, and everyone, including the lost individual, had an observer controller close by for safety who knew where he was but could not reveal it. Said another way, the individual was in no real harm because we would not have let anything fire above his head, but the pressure of constant heat and the bombardment of questions added to the pressure, which made it a perfect training event.

Over the years, however, I've laughed less, and I've concluded that many of us fall into the category of not knowing where we are. All of us tend to look up and somehow assume our point of reference can be seen by all when, in truth, it can't. We should all simply admit the truth: "I'm lost." I know I've been there!

As we look at our nation after the COVID crisis and see the ads pop up for mental health awareness, I think it's important to acknowledge that we are all sometimes lost and need assistance. Those who put off admitting alcoholism, drug addiction, sex addiction, gambling, etc., hurt others as much as themselves. Those who make false accusations are equally liable.

- *Tell me about a time you were under the cloud that looks like a duck. Did others laugh or come to your aid? What did you learn? What will you do when others need your help?*

Put The Damn Phone Down

Ah, a nice family walk.

Sitting on my deck in Grand County, Colorado, I see something that warms my heart: families taking morning and evening walks. Fido or Sparky leads, sniffing every bush and leaving their mark at every tree. Junior and Suzie are running along talking, yet they are not even paying enough attention to see if anyone is listening. And, ah, here come Mom and Dad, taking up the rear of the family formation. How wonderful it is to see a complete family enjoying the mountain fresh air provided by nature. I know that much of the hardship COVID brought on will be overshadowed by the goodness of those kids, finally seeing Mom and Dad walking with them. Yes, COVID was and still is horrible; the isolation kept us at home. People couldn't physically go to work, so families had to stay home, play with their kids, and even take family walks. Dads now play with kids, having tea parties with their nine-year-olds at 9 a.m. in the living room, followed by a board meeting with the forty-nine-year-olds on Zoom at 10 a.m. It was one of the few good things that came out of this horrible time.

Being a father of three and a former infantry soldier, I rarely had the opportunity to work from home in my twenty-six years of service. However, when I was able, I did play with my kids, and fortunately, at the time they were growing up, cell phones were not as popular. We loved playing a version of Cooper softball. All it took was a tennis ball, a plastic bat, and three jackets, one for each base. The kids all lined up behind each other. I was both the pitcher and all the basemen. Once the kids got up to bat and got a hit, they ran around all the bases, touching each jacket with their foot while I chased them with the ball, hoping to tag them out. We played this game for over three years when they were in elementary school. I never caught them, and they always won. A simple game with a tennis ball that a dog had previously chewed, an old plastic bat, and our jackets made for the most memorable times ever.

Recently, however, what I saw during the COVID crisis as families took walks has disturbed me. I've seen wonderful families walking, but some were carrying this annoying crutch called a cell phone. So yes, you have the perfect family, except the parents in the back are talking on their phones, obviously not paying attention to anything. Now, let me give those parents taking up the rear some advice.

Put the damn phone down; better yet, leave it at home. I can't tell you the number of times I've seen kids without parents because both parents, albeit being geographically present, are chatting on the damn phone. Yes, I know it was not your intention to talk while walking with Junior and Suzie, but your best friend from college, the boss from work, or your mom called. Well, guess what? If you left your phone at home, there would be a missed call, and you could call them back.

CHAPTER 2

Oh, you think, "I'm carrying it for safety." What if a moose or bear runs toward you? Well, if you think a phone will help, then good luck. Let me play this scenario:

"Ahh!"

"911, what is your emergency?"

"Ah, I'm being attacked by a bear!"

"Okay, we will dispatch a unit; they should be there in ten minutes."

The truth is if you weren't on your damn phone, you would have probably not walked up to the bear. And if you think a bear is going to hang around for ten minutes after mauling your ass, well, you're wrong. I also don't think the thirty minutes you're gone for a walk are going to make a life-or-death situation worse. What about, "I have a nine o'clock conference call I need to take?" Okay, take the 9 a.m. conference call at home, leave the phone at the desk when you're done, and walk at 10 a.m. Look, I know you are an important VP or CEO, but you know what? If you dropped dead tomorrow, the company would still run just fine, so what's thirty minutes without office gossip? And oh, by the way, if the company or your department is so fragile that it would fall apart if you were not on your phone all the time, then truthfully, you have failed the most important task a leader can have: to train your subordinates.

So, for thirty minutes a day, don't be a babysitter; be a parent, walk with your kids, and be sure to pick up Fido's mess when he poops in my yard. Find out what's on your kid's mind, and when your kid or your partner starts to drive you crazy, walk alone. But don't forget Fido, because if you do need to talk, dogs, except for Siberian huskies and beagles, never talk back; they are the model for listening.

I know that it sounds harsh, but take it from someone who missed every one of his kids' first steps, who missed the training wheels, who missed numerous sporting events, who missed school recognition events, and who missed three proms. The job is just not worth it. Plan your schedule around your family, and if you can't because the boss is an asshole, simply fire your boss by quitting your job.

- *Take a minute and go look at your kids: If they are in sixth grade, they will be out of the house in six years. If they are in high school, they will be gone before the stock option you just received vests. Time is critical. Kids will never remember the stock option or the new truck, but they will remember the walk they took with you and Fido. I want you to put the phone down and go on a walk with your family. Write me a note and tell me how it felt.*

Is It Best To Be An Owl Or A Sled Dog?

Growing up in Alaska, I experienced firsthand the appeal of adventure. Books like *The Glacier Pilot*, *The Flying North*, and *Wager with the Wind* told harrowing stories of famous pilots who made Alaska what it is today: a haven for bush pilots. Because in Alaska there are only three highways, for most who live there, traveling by air is not a luxury but a requirement.

I didn't just read about flying; I also read about the Klondike gold rush and bear attacks. If it was about Alaska, I read it. One book that stuck out was Jack London's *The Call of the Wild*. London wrote many books, each highlighting the plight and struggles of early Alaska and the Yukon Territory. I was fascinated with *The Call of the Wild*, especially with Buck, the famous dog who was the main character. By the way, the book is much better than the movie.

I became so captivated by the book in my early years that I would travel downtown to watch the Fur Rendezvous parade. Seeing all the dog sled teams fascinated me.

I often think back to those times and realize just how lucky I really was to experience so much at such a young age.

Recently, I saw an ad for eyeglasses as I watched my nightly hour of news. I became engrossed by this commercial; it showed an owl wearing glasses having a conversation with a young lady. At first, I was confused, as owls are known for having the best vision, except eagles, so why would an owl have glasses? Secondly, I was wondering why an intelligent-looking girl was having a conversation with the owl. Regardless, it's a commercial, right? Probably made by the same company that shows dogs driving cars.

At that point, I asked myself, Would I rather be an owl or a sled dog? Owls can turn their heads 180 degrees and have perfect vision, but sled dogs are strong and dependable. The owl sits on a perch and observes; it represents a real bystander like me. Owls get a view with no one to answer to. They are accountable, responsible, and able to pick and choose what they want to do. It was then clear that as a civilian, I had been a sled dog for too long. When I was in the lead, I was tied to the reins. When I was part of the team, the only thing I saw was the assholes of the lead dogs.

I now recognize that my previous experiences were worse than wearing a mask. My life was like having a mask with cellophane over my head; not only was I misrepresenting who I was, but I could not breathe to become who I am. Somehow many of us fool ourselves into thinking that we can be both an owl and a sled dog, but I don't think we can. Businesses love slogans that show cooperation, trust, and free thinking. Well, that slogan works during the job interview and maybe a month later, but as any seasoned executive will tell you, culture eats strategy for lunch every day. If you don't fit into the culture, you're gone; there is no in-between.

CHAPTER 2

I have taken the cellophane and the mask off so I can see, be seen for who I am, and breathe.

Yes, I am no longer a sled dog confined by the drama of looking straight ahead and following; I am now an owl able to see and be part of all the dreams around me.

- *Think about your day. When could you benefit by being a sled dog? When do you think the perspective of an owl would help? What are you doing to change?*

The Revolving Door

Sometimes I see myself as a failure, sometimes as a success, and sometimes I lie at the crossroads of indecision.

I often look at others and compare myself using their model of what I want or don't want to be. Unlike Dr. Seuss, I let those who did not matter in my life have a vote. I've even used well-accepted metrics to show my achievements and then put together a to-do list to fill in the areas I'm deficient in.

I allowed others to define who I was and what I should do, thereby almost guaranteeing I'd be a failure or a constant follower—very much the same thing in my book. When I was feeling down, I would look at the similarities on the list I created as an antidote to pick me up. Whenever I was feeling good, I would revert to what I had not done to bring me back to Earth. This was my whirlpool moment, my continuous sine curve of emotions.

I now ask the questions, "Was my life embodied? Did I give myself to my beliefs? Did I incorporate spirituality?" And the answer, every time, is a resounding no.

I've now transitioned from defining myself using lists and metrics made by others to recreating myself using the revolving door. I am focused on who I am first and foremost, tossing the mask of conformity in the trash.

CHAPTER 2

- *Outside of the workplace, how often have you defined yourself based on metrics others have described? When are you going to change?*

Mind To Heart

For some reason, what's on my mind today is the word "escape." I want to get away, away from it all. I long for a walk into the wilderness, as the Israelites did in the Bible. I just want to escape, as Polish popstar Basia says in her song "Miles Away." In both cases, it's about escaping into nature.

Perhaps that's why, when I'm flying, I'm in my element; it's my escape, my world. As I travel at one hundred and thirty-five knots through McClure Pass or over Castle Peak, I no longer worry about my engine quitting. I now worry about what really matters, like the "engine" on top of my neck quitting. How can I embrace going with the flow?

The wind coming over one peak and down the other makes for a turbulent ride, much like giving in to one's emotions.

As I work on my getaway, my escape, I find it's about the ranch I'd like to buy in Routt County, Colorado, or the log cabin in Alaska. My escape is all within me and within my capability.

My movement from confinement to freedom has everything to do with the transition from my mind to my heart—eighteen of the longest inches in the world.

- *When was the last time you wanted to escape? Where did you go?*

CHAPTER 2

- *Tell me how you managed your eighteen-inch journey from mind to heart? What were some of the roadblocks?*

Chapter 3

Nature

When I wrote this chapter, our nation was paralyzed by the COVID pandemic. People were locked in their homes, afraid to go outside, with thermometers at the ready near each entry. Bringing packages in from the outside only to let them sit for a day because we wanted to ensure there was time for the COVID germs to die. Seeing neighbors in the street, only to wave and walk in the other direction. Saying goodbye to our loved ones who were ill through a pane of glass at the hospital or nursing home with an iPad held by a wonderful first-line worker we hardly knew. What horror we all faced and went through. I applaud the work done by both US administrations to get us out of this dilemma. We had the world's best and brightest working and successfully developing a vaccine at warp speed, something never done before.

I was one of those who isolated themselves. I went to a place of solitude, a place the size of Rhode Island yet with a population of less than 16,000. I went and lived within the confines of nature at 8,700 feet above sea level in the Rocky Mountains of Colorado. Before you comment on how lucky I was, I will be vulnerable, and tell you that I also suffered like many other Americans. I broke up with the person I had dated for five years, I lost my mom to colon cancer, and I was completely separated from my three adult kids. I was lonely, sad, and sad for others like me. To top it off, I, like millions of others, also contracted COVID in September 2020, prior to a vaccine coming out.

As I went through this transition of solitude that all of us were experiencing, I adopted a rhythm to incorporate and appreciate what was immediately around me—a rhythm I now can't do without: nature. I made time to sit each morning to enjoy what is already with us, already free, so fulfilling. Ironically, it took tragedy for me to recognize the greatness of nature and appreciate what was always around me. It took God to make me so tired that all I had energy for was to look. It took losing the one I loved, who loved to walk, loved to look at the simple leaves, and loved to sit outside, to recognize how essential all those things were and what I should have done while she was still in my life. It took losing my mom, someone I did not call enough, see enough, or have the courage to tell how much I loved when we spoke, to understand that all of us have limited time on this Earth, and we need to learn not only to love ourselves but to love others and tell them we love them.

This chapter highlights the aspects of nature that caused me to take off my mask of conformity and urgency. The chapter highlights thoughts while looking at nature and what matters in the Dr. Seuss dialogue, something we can all appreciate.

Ten minutes of appreciating nature each day, whether it be a tree in your backyard, a bush at the city park, or the rain hitting the cars in the parking lot, will make you wonder why you haven't done it before, and those ten minutes will soon become twenty or even thirty.

Each morning when I wake up, I walk downstairs and look out the window, and every morning I see something different. This routine has forced me to put down the many things I used to carry in my arms, on my shoulders, and in my mind. It forced me to finally understand what my dad had shown me years ago, that the most important things in life are not things.

As Susan McHenry said, "Everyone is bald beneath their hair." Well, my hair came off when COVID hit, and I'm now exposing my baldness to each of you.

I hope you get several things from this chapter:
- *The joy your current surroundings bring.*
- *The journey of enjoying nature is more important than any destination and that journey could even be called a destination.*

We Are All Just Snowflakes

There are two things I can watch and never become bored with: snow falling and my fireplace. Both are mesmerizing and relaxing and provide immense comfort.

As I watch the snow fall, I sometimes look out as far as I can see and try to find a flake of snow to follow on its short trajectory from the base of the low clouds to the ground. I think of how the flake was formed, probably at ten thousand feet or higher, and how it made it through the clouds, being battered around by the wind and other flakes, to appear before my eyes and settle on a structure, a tree, or the ground to blend in and provide needed moisture. I think about the journey that little flake must have gone through to make it to the Earth, and then I think about how many flakes did not make it to the Earth.

This thought leads me to my journey and our journey. In a way, aren't we all like snowflakes? We start life in the womb and enter the world, where some of us have a tough upbringing.

As we get stronger and older, we take on a defined shape, using what our parents taught us, what we learned in school, our social environment, and finally our corporate culture. Like the wind battering the snow as it shapes each flake, our environment shapes us. We climb that ladder toward our dream, like the snowflake making its way to the ground, each headed to destiny as moisture or ash.

But let's not stop there, because while that snowflake is falling to provide moisture needed in the ground for us to sustain life, our work on Earth needs to be equally providing. We need to ensure our priorities are God, our family, and our community. While we may get battered in our jobs, in our neighborhoods, and within our environment, in the end we need to keep our focus, so when our time on Earth ends, and it will end, we will have made the difference God put us here to make. Just like a snowflake.

- *What similarities do you see between your journey and the snowflake's?*

- *How will you ensure your personal ground is nourished and you've made the difference you were put here to make before going to heaven?*

The Berthoud Pass Lesson Of Life

I was reading an article by my good friend Frosty Woolridge, a well-known author of seventeen books. Many of his articles are about his travels and life on six continents. This article, though, was about the happiness factor and was a short comparison of life in Bhutan and the US. While reading and agreeing with Frosty's findings, I was struck by the passage: "How fast do we really need to go to get there?"[8]

The mechanical part of me quickly said, "It depends on how much time you have." My anti-heart, sometimes called my brain, quickly did some calculations to lead me to believe that the speed needed to arrive at my destination on time is a factor of the distance and my time available to travel. So, if I have an hour to travel sixty miles, I need to go sixty miles per hour to get where I am going. Or better yet, if I only have fifty minutes, I need to go seventy miles per hour, and then I have an excuse to go fast, right?

But wait, Frosty said, "How fast do we really need to go to get there?" There was no time constraint, so why did I allow my anti-heart to put a time constraint in?

My mind says if we need to be there by a certain time, a time that requires us to go fast, go straight, and not pay attention to the journey. Hmmm, but isn't the journey part of the fun? I mean, if we were on the Starship Enterprise, then we could go to the transporter room

---

[8] Frosty Wooldridge (speaker, author, environmentalist, patriot), www.frostywooldridge.com, 2022.

and get beamed anywhere, right? But we don't have a transporter room; we have roads, communities along those roads, and people in those communities, and there are potential memories we could make with those people in those communities. So, except in an emergency, if we solely focus on getting there, then maybe we should not go at all. Frosty's point, so well stated, is that "It's not the miles you make, it's the pictures, conversations, and spiritual awakening along thc way."

It took me fifty years to realize I could never have any meaningful engagement by going fast. I spent the first six years of my life in elementary school, and I can still name each of my teachers and recall what they looked like, especially Ms. Williams, my 4th grade teacher, whom I had a crush on. It traumatized me when, one day in 1969, right before class ended, a man walked in who she introduced to the class as her fiancé. It took me years to get over that heartache.

Ironically, I can relate to and identify with so many things in my life during my early years because I took things slow. But as I got older, I moved faster without regard to looking around and understanding the environment. Looking back, I should have slowed down, regardless of the outside pressure to move up.

As I now sit in my home in Grand County, Colorado, I sometimes reminisce on my travels up and down Berthoud Pass. Some drivers don't like Berthoud Pass, as it can be intimidating given the sharp curves combined with steep ascents and descents. But Berthoud Pass is a wonderful drive if you pay attention to the road and not your cell phone. Its beauty is unmatched, and the Colorado road crews keep the pass in great shape. The pass teaches every driver an important, lifelong lesson. Going up the hill, there are two lanes. You can pass, jockey in and out, and even stop to take a picture. The lanes are wide and offer options. But once you reach the summit of the pass, there is only one lane down. Regardless of how fast you made it up the hill, you're only going to go as fast as the person in front of you down the hill. Isn't that what life teaches us? There is a point in life when, no matter how fast you make it up, there is usually only one way down.

For now, let's think about living where we are with who we are, and when we do venture out, let's enjoy the journey to our destination and take the urgency mask off. God knows, my friend Frosty gets an A+ for always abiding by and living by that belief; I am now one of his faithful students.

- *Think of a time you were in such a hurry you missed the scenery along the way only to hear about it from someone who took their time.*
- *Frosty's windshield is much bigger than his rear-view mirror. Tell me about your windshield. What are you doing to make it even bigger?*

Watching Nature Rest

The sunlight hits the opposite hill like a big spotlight during a Broadway play. The air is still, the leaves are green, and the lodgepole trees stand at peace. It is Grand County, and it is morning. It's fifty-five degrees, and even the mosquitoes have yet to wake up. There is a peace in the wilderness that transcends all. Everyone and everything must rest. I find it such an honor to be awake or, better yet, to awaken to watch nature rest. I now know I was made restless by God to get up and watch nature rest.

Now, I will join nature and go back to sleep.

- *Everything must rest, and sometimes you can feel peace from watching others rest. Remember the feeling you got after a long day's work when you walked into a loved one's room to see them sound asleep, not a worry in the world, because you are their keeper? Tell me what that felt like.*
- *When was the last time you got up to watch nature rest? Wasn't it the same peaceful feeling as watching your loved one sleep?*

The Smudge

As I was eating my breakfast one morning, I looked out at the vast forest that's around my home—the sea of never-ending trees. I saw birds fly and the snow fall like the dust of an angel in a Disney movie. Then suddenly I saw—wait, what is that? Is it a smudge on the window? How the heck did that happen?

Who would've put a smudge on my perfect window? Was it inside or out? Asking this question was key because then I could assign blame for my discomfort, and we know how important blame is, right? Not.

My entire breakfast was now sitting on the table, getting cold, while I got Windex to clean the smudge. After seeing the smudge was not on the inside but on the outside, I felt better because there's no way I could've caused it. So, I sat back down, said my prayers, ate my moderately warm sausage and eggs, and took my lukewarm coffee to the microwave, only to turn my head back to stare at the smudge I had no control over and did not cause.

After sitting down, my eyes no longer focused on the beauty of the trees, the vastness of the forest, or the snow, but on the smudge. The distraction of the smudge took away the meaning and beauty of everything around me.

I then thought, how often have I been distracted, not by smudges but by things that did not really make a difference? How often have I let meaningless things have meaning?

The next time your partner, child, or subordinate does something you question or the house has a pile of laundry on the floor, remember to see the beauty of your loved ones and friends and embrace the warmth of your home. Start by looking through the entire window, or even through a different window, and find the goodness in what you are looking at through the window. Instead of complaining, take your partner and hold their hand. Trust me, the laundry will wait, and the smudge, even if you wipe it off, there will be plenty more.

- *Look outside through your windows. Do you notice the smudge or the beauty provided by God?*
- *Now look at your partner. Do you see the extra ten pounds on their waist (a synonym for the smudge), or do you see that spark in their eyes that caused you to fall in love with them? Tell me about that spark and why it's so wonderful.*

The Importance Of The Deck

I was sitting at my dining room table one day, eating breakfast while looking at the beautiful mountains surrounding me. The sunshine was glorious, making the glittering snow shine through my windows, which made me realize just how dirty my windows were.

Each one I looked at had this film I could probably write my name in. You know, like the "wash me" we so often see on automobiles? I then wondered what beauty I was missing due to the dirty film obstructing my view.

At that point, my eye began to itch, probably because I was speaking of "looking," so I took off my glasses to scratch my eyelid. As I put my glasses on, I was embarrassed. Man, they were also filthy.

So I pondered for a minute. I have the most beautiful view of nature outside my backyard, and I am looking through dirty windows and dirty eyeglasses. What have I missed? What else is out there?

As we look at our own environment, sometimes we are taken aback by things because the lens we view things through is obstructed or distorted—whether it be friends saying what they think of someone you love, a teacher explaining something about your child, or an associate at work discussing office politics. The point being, to get a fair perspective, you must wash your lens.

As in my house, I've learned that when I really want to get a clear view—a view not distorted by dirty windows and glasses, a view where my eyes can be the direct reflection from the conduit of my heart, a real unobstructed view—then sometimes it's best to go outside past the windows, take off the glasses, sit on the deck, and look. A deck where you don't have to worry about the windows to clean, a deck where you no longer need glasses to see, a deck where you can just be.

- *What's causing your distorted view in life? The news? Your social media? What are you doing to move away from it all and go to your deck?*
- *How will you know when you're there?*
- *What are you going to do to remain there?*

Different Views

For years, every morning I made a four-cup pot of coffee. As the coffee brewed, I religiously abided by my no-media rule and refused to touch or look at my phone or call anyone during this early quiet time of mine. This was my time. As the last drops of coffee entered the decanter, I quickly pulled the carafe out, only to hear the final drops sizzle on a hot burner while I poured my first cup of coffee.

I would walk into the living room and sit in my favorite chair to view the picturesque Rocky Mountains through my windows, taking a moment to truly grasp the beauty around me. After several minutes, I changed my position to get a different view. I would treasure the beauty, then finish my coffee and move onto what was to be my day.

One day, I had a guest. That person got up before me, and when I came down, they were sitting in my favorite chair. Oh boy, can you believe that someone would have the nerve to sit in my favorite chair? That chair is my Archie Bunker chair!

I smiled and said good morning, and we started chatting. After making and serving her coffee, I went to a different part of the living room, my couch, so I could see her as we engaged in conversation. She was mesmerized, as I was, by the beauty of the outside. And as she talked, my listening skills diminished, for my focus was more on the outside than our conversation.

Ironically, it was because of her sitting in the chair I always did that I was in this new space that was the couch. This new space gave me a view I'd never seen. It was very much the same perspective I got when taking my conformity mask off—a view that opened my eyes and heart to a new beauty of nature.

Sometimes we all need to change seats to see what we're missing and what matters.

- *Think about what would change in your life if you could view it from a different perspective.*
- *For those of you who have a favorite chair, pick an evening when no one else is around and sit somewhere else. What do you feel? What do you see?*

I Observe

The green pastures across the way are replaced by a white blanket, looking like a lumpy comforter as it follows the contours of the ground. The lodgepole trees standing erect look like Christmas trees. The moon is still visible. There is no wind, and the raven seeking an early meal flies in front of me as I watch it from one window to the next. The branch struggles as it tries to support the snow. It now bends like a spoon holding a brick, resembling the Big Dipper. I no longer stare; I no longer look. For now, I am at peace and enjoy harmony.

It's not Christmas; it's not even winter. It's Easter 2020, and once again it snowed in Grand County, Colorado. As we are locked in, unable to attend the traditional Easter Service due to the pandemic, and unable to see our friends and loved ones, we observe that God knows no bounds when it comes to showing His true beauty. And He reminds us of His beautiful, unpredictable nature by blessing us with a big snow in the spring.

- *God has a mysterious way of giving the confidence to the trees that when they shed their leaves, they're going to come back. He gives equal confidence to the snow, that it will nourish the ground.*
- *God surprised us with a loving blanket of snow this Easter. Who will you surprise to let them know how much you love them and to let them know you will come back?*

Shedding The Mask Of Comparison

During my morning sit in my favorite chair, I always look through one particular pane of glass that, through restrictions based on the size and shape of the window, only allows me to see three branches of a mighty lodgepole tree outside.

When I first started this tradition, it was winter, and all the branches were bare, with no blooms, blossoms, or leaves. Randomly, I chose the center branch and said to myself, "That branch represents me." I thought I would follow its progression through the winter, and as it blossomed, I would blossom, too.

Well, as spring came and the other branches showed promise of bloom, my branch was bare. My branch will bloom a little later, I thought. I'll catch up. Then came summer, and while the other branches had a solid green growth of buds, my branch had just one bud.

For months, I thought, well, maybe this comparison is a snapshot of my life: always behind, not picked as the first string. Now that I am sixty, I realize that catching up is a synonym for skepticism and comparing myself to others. I choose to no longer be a hostage to hate, skepticism, or acknowledgment that others are better. I decided that the time was now to stop following and start holding myself accountable.

At sixty, I was determined to change my view, and I did. At sixty, I choose not to be what something or someone else is but to be appreciative of who I am. And

CHAPTER 3

I'm damn sure I'm not second to anyone or anything.

- *Sit back and put this book on your lap. Think about what you are doing or going to do to change your view. How long will that take?*
- *What's blocking your view? Why?*

What Is Our Destiny?

I watched *The Call of the Wild* for the second time. Somehow movies always seem better after the first viewing because you notice things you missed the first time around. Toward the end of the movie, the lead character, played by Harrison Ford, is sitting on a hill overlooking the woods. He tells his dog, Buck (the protagonist), "This is timber wolf country." About three minutes later, you see a herd of caribou running through the woods like a stampede chased by a pack of timber wolves. Hmm, I thought.

It reminded me of the wild animal shows I used to watch portraying African wildlife, especially the wildebeests crossing the Nile River at the same locations each year as the many crocodiles waited with anticipation. It's half-eerie and half-entertaining to see the wildebeests stop at the shoreline and look the crocodiles deep in the eye for what seems like an eternity. I often wonder what they're saying to each other.

"Hey, you know we cross here every year, right?" says the wildebeest.

"Yep," says the crocodile.

"So, try to only eat twelve of us this year; we have a couple of young ones in the herd we really need to get across."

"Roger that," says the crocodile. "I'll pass the request along."

CHAPTER 3

Part of me wants to fly to Africa and erect a bridge across the Nile River to see if the wildebeests will continue to cross through the river or use my bridge. In my case, whether a caribou or wildebeest, the why sets in. Why do animals knowingly expose themselves to danger, fully aware that some members of the herd will ultimately die?

Well, I've concluded that it's not habit or stupidity. It's destiny. The prey and the predator have unique roles. Each has a destiny.

As humans, what is our destiny? Is it a path set by others? Is it as firm as railroad tracks? Is it an open field so we can change direction at each obstacle?

So, what could have been our destiny is now a traffic circle. What was once known is now unknown. What was once expected is now a surprise. Nature has no ego, animals have no ego, animals have no traffic circle, animals don't seek the approval of anyone, and they do just fine, given the human predator does not interfere.

Maybe it's time we joined Buck and Harrison Ford's character on that hill and re-examined our destiny as human beings from nature's point of view. Maybe it's time we let fear and ego go by the wayside and let God take His course. Animals don't have masks, so why should we?

- *If one believes eternal life is possible, then what are we denying ourselves by deflecting our destiny?*

Present, No Longer Just Passing Through

In my senior year of college, I bought a Turbo Trans Am. It had a big emblem of an eagle on the hood, a T-top, and a cassette deck, which allowed me to play the best tunes, predominantly Boston, Marvin Gaye, and Ray Parker Jr. When the weather was nice, I was in T-top heaven, letting the air rush through my half-inch afro as I cruised along Interstate 87 headed toward New York City on weekends. My next car, a 280ZX, was even faster and came with the recorded voice of a sexy lady who let me know my door was open or fuel was low. I called her Sexy Suzy.

Finally, after two years of paying for expensive gas along with speeding tickets, I sold my fast car and bought a truck with an AM radio and no air conditioning. At the time, I lived in Kansas, a state that had both humidity and tremendous heat.

I soon realized that because I no longer had a T-top to enjoy the sun while driving, I had to stop and get out to enjoy the countryside. So after about twenty years, the year I came back home from Iraq, I reached deep into my pockets and bought a convertible coupe. I loved driving through the countryside with the top down. After realizing that the wind that hit my head was getting colder each time, primarily because I was getting bald, I no longer lowered the top and later sold the car. A short time later, yep, you guessed it, I bought a truck—this time a four-door 4x4 with air conditioning.

Now, after the COVID lockdown and after

appreciating the wonder of slowing down, sitting, and walking, I no longer crave the convertible or the T-top. Now when the days are nice, I drive my truck with the radio turned on, and when I see something that catches my attention, I stop and get out, look up at the sky, and soak in the goodness of my surroundings. I have transitioned from taking the top off and driving to stopping and being present.

- *Take a second and think of your transition. Where has it taken you?*
- *Are you present or just passing through?*

Raton Pass: The Gateway To America's Past

My nine-year-old truck Rufus and I were going through Trinidad, Colorado, on I-25, headed over to Raton Pass, elevation 7,835 feet. (As a little side note, my truck was named Sweetie Pie until I hit a deer and the grill was damaged to the point it looked like the mouth of a hockey player, so I changed the name of my truck from Sweetie Pie to Rufus.)

Another mountain pass, another windy, curvy adventure. For someone who lives on the other side of a mountain pass and travels through mountain passes every week, there was something different about this one: Travel through this pass was quick.

When I got to the top, I didn't see curves headed down. I saw the other side; I saw America; I saw John Wayne's Western plateau; I saw the purple sky and majestic light; I saw the wagon trains of the 1800s as they proceeded toward the Spanish Peaks. I thought of the beautiful rendition of Ray Charles singing "America" and the inspirational Lee Greenwood singing "Proud to Be an American." Raton Pass may be just 7,835 feet, but it is the gateway to America.

- *Nature has a funny way of opening our eyes, sometimes causing us to pay tribute to our own history.*
- *When was the last time you looked out the window and visualized the history of what that location once was?*

What Does Silence Sound Like?

When I am at peace, I often sit and look out, not staring at anything, just looking. Because, to me, the observation of being still is sometimes more exciting than action. So, I wondered, if asked about moments of peace, stillness, and silence, how would I describe them?

When we eat, we compare food if we don't know how to describe it. The first time I had a meal containing alligator in Leesville, Louisiana, I told others it tasted like chicken.

But to sit in silence is more along the lines of what you don't hear. Sitting in silence means finally understanding what silence sounds like. You are in a trance, where you are sleeping with your eyes wide open and your brain is unaware of anything. You are sitting without judgment, as some would say. You're just sitting. Maybe Simon and Garfunkel had it right with their sixties hit "The Sound of Silence." How will we know when we are hearing silence? How will we know the Sound of Silence?

- *Think about your life. What are you doing to recognize silence? Better yet, what are you doing to really enjoy the silence once it's recognized?*
- *What will it take for all of us to appreciate silence more?*

Twelve Minutes On A Path To My Purpose

It's 4:42 a.m., the sky is light, the wind is calm, COVID is rampant, and I am in Alaska. I often think about the pioneers who discovered and formed this wonderful state and how, with limited knowledge and resources, they navigated through pandemics and epidemics.

I could start by looking at the leaders from the early 1900s who led our nation through the Spanish flu. I could then move forward to the great WWII veterans; what would they do if they were in charge now? What if we had leaders in the Senate like the late Ted Stevens, a Republican, and Daniel Inouye, a Democrat, both of whom focused on one solution: a better America? Or even Presidents Kennedy or Reagan? How would they have handled this pandemic?

It's now 4:54 a.m. Twelve minutes have passed. The beauty of nature remains, but my purpose is now found. I now know I'm the one to make a difference; I can no longer continue to point fingers and watch the news. It's time to get off my ass; that's why I'm here. As Abraham Lincoln once said, "It's the life in your years, not the years in your life," and I have a lot of life left in my years.

- *What changed in your life as you went through COVID?*
- *How did that change affect your life?*

The Foreplay Of Fog

Wow, look at that beautiful hill! With the tree branches glistening and the sun trying to peek through openings between branches, I can see a Minnesota Christmas tree farm with every evergreen perfectly arranged. I then look out my window to the south at the tall lodgepole trees—so tall, so far, yet so close. It seems as if I can grab one and shimmy down to the frozen Earth like a fireman's pole.

Then a small cloud separates from a large bank of clouds in the distance. It moves like a kid running away from his parents at Disney World, and in an instant, like the guy sitting in front of you at a concert, his head (the cloud) blocks the most beautiful view of the hill I just had. I try to see through it; I move my head to the left, then to the right, still to no avail. Why did that cloud choose the hill I was looking at to settle on top of?

Then, it's as though the cloud had called his buddies, and more small clouds appear, and like LEGO blocks, they all connect and form a fog, so what was once my beautiful, glistening view has now become a gray afterthought. But wait, I think I start to see the trees in the distance once again! Oh good, another cloud moved out of the way, and I'm starting to get my view back. Maybe it will clear up soon and the fog will dissipate; maybe it won't, and that will be okay, too. Regardless, I know what's behind the fog. It's a beautiful view. Just as you know, the sun is still shining even on the cloudiest of days.

- *How will you adjust your thoughts, so you see the inner beauty in everyday life regardless if there is fog or someone's big head blocks your view?*

The Darkness Of Anger Overcome By The Light Of God

I tossed and turned all night; I just couldn't sleep. I finally got up, went downstairs at 5:39 a.m., and sat, only to stare into the darkness. The silence is interrupted by the sound of one truck on the road, and then once again, there is silence. Why couldn't I sleep? Well, I was bitter. I was thinking of how all the great American companies were losing so many good people who made such a wonderful difference in the companies' successes. How these workers had missed soccer games or first communions just to ensure the company they worked for was running smoothly.

What I was witnessing was companies letting people go like cattle because of COVID. I get it; it's about revenue and sales, and you know what? The easiest way to improve the next quarter's numbers is to lay people off. But most of those employees must pay for their house, braces, kids' soccer uniforms, and many other bills; sometimes what is easy is not always the best.

That's why God woke me up. Those were not healthy thoughts, and God wanted me to know He had other plans for me.

For the second time in a week, God let me know that bitterness and anger were not acceptable. God, I get it, I thought, and I admit that forgiveness is just a bit hard to accept when I look around me and see people who are so financially affected by this pandemic.

I then looked up at the twenty-one windowpanes that face south in my house, trying to see, as I do every day, what had changed about the scenery outside my windows, but it was still dark. I glanced over one windowpane to the left and saw two stars—stars so bright they looked like flashlights shining through my windows.

As I continued to stare, the stars appeared to be moving closer together.

What was God trying to tell me? Did the stars represent a relationship? Me coming closer to someone? Was it a sign of destiny to wake me up only to say, quit staring and start looking? Was it a sign that the people initially affected by this pandemic and job loss would be okay?

As morning crept in, the darkness faded and the room got a bit lighter; I could no longer see the stars, and the tree I normally watched was hardly visible. To top it off, it was now completely cloudy. How in the world could I see two stars just an hour ago during the morning darkness, and now it's so cloudy I can hardly see the tree in front of the house?

I surmised that God got me up to see what was coming my way through the clouds and the trees. God wanted me to know that sometimes we see our best in total darkness and that the darkness of anger sometimes blocks our view. God wanted me to stop staring and start looking. God saw through the bitterness I could not see through to tell me there was a brighter future for all, and all I needed to do was have faith.

CHAPTER 3

- *How many things in your life are so close to you that you're missing the bigger picture?*
- *When was the last time you woke up earlier than planned? What was on your mind? What was God telling you?*

The Penetrating Glow Of Sunrise

"The night is darkest right before the dawn." [9]

As I rise each morning, I'm struck by the glow of sunlight piercing the night sky as it tries to get through my windows to my bedroom. The journey that a ray of sunlight must cut through in the winter sky to reach my window and land on my comforter must be tough. So, as those rays pierce all the cold air and travel through the window and the glass doors of my bedroom to my comforter, I do what others are known to do—I pull it over my head so as to reside in the comfort of darkness once again.

As time passes, that comforter no longer blocks the sun. I need something a bit thicker, so I reach for the trusty thick pillow; it's like armor when it comes to ensuring darkness.

Why, when God is clearly trying to get me up, am I continuing to hide even though I am not asleep? I am, in my own way, still secluded in my world of darkness. It's time I acknowledge, not hide from, the glow of sunrise and apply that glow as one of my many life's lessons.

What is it about life that we tend to run from? Why is it that when nature knocks on our door, we tend to hide? Whether or not we can see the sun on cloudy days is irrelevant; it's always there, and in someone's

---

[9] Sir Thomas Fuller, *A Pisgah Sight of Palestine and the Confines Thereof* (1869).

life, somewhere, it will shine.

Perhaps when people try to do nice things for you, or perhaps when you are being comforted, you should remove your pillow and your comforter and just smile to welcome their warmth as you would welcome the penetrating glow of the sun.

- *When in your life has God tried to wake you up, only to have you hide again? What were you hiding from? Are you still hiding?*
- *Think of the last time you snapped at someone who had good meaning to help you. How did it feel? They were just trying to bring some light into your life like the sun was piercing my sheet, pillow, and comforter. Next time, move all the obstacles and welcome their actions with a smile, and I guarantee you'll have a much better day.*

Chapter 4

Moving Toward God, Learning To Love Myself

But the fig tree said unto them, "Should I forsake my sweetness, and my good fruit, and go to be promoted over the trees?" (Judges 9:11).

This was a great chapter to write, as it highlighted most of the things I have done wrong in my life. As per the passage above, I had forsaken my individual fruitfulness by stepping away from God. My mask of societal conformity was being replaced by a mask of allegiance to God. It was interesting to be able to look at where and why I failed. Many times, I followed tracks laid by others. Other times, I was just wandering, walking by sight, not faith—the opposite of what 2 Corinthians 5:7 tells us to do.

During my journey of writing this chapter, I learned some important things:

- *Being kind is more important than being right.*
- *I will be driven no longer by reputation but by purpose.*
- *Sometimes our mess is a message.*

As you read these stories, you will see a range of emotions spanning from anger and sadness to

CHAPTER 4

contentment. This was a hard journey for me, and, in truth, it still is. But the saving grace was my realization that to really be the person I needed to be, I had to love myself first.

I hope you enjoy it.

Our Daughters

One week, I went to visit my two daughters, who live in Texas. Both left home about the same time, yet they are five years apart. Now they are on their own, in two cities in the same state. I'm the one who travels to see them; I'm now the one who misses them. They have their whole lives ahead of them, and just like when they were little, I constantly worry about them. Who will they meet, who will keep them safe, and what will they ultimately do?

I'm hopeful yet scared that they'll meet someone like me. For all the love I have for them, I was not the best husband to my wife—I sometimes got angry, yet I could never envision anyone yelling at my daughters. I was not the best customer in a restaurant, demanding things that were trivial like salsa or barbecue sauce, only to see a waitress trying to meet not only my needs but the many needs of other self-serving customers.

At times during my many travels, I would often sit in first class, only to watch other men treat female flight attendants as objects, wanting two to three drinks prior to taking off. So why do I want my daughters to meet someone like me? Well, because I'm no longer the guy I used to be.

I wish when I got mad at my girlfriends, I could see the disappointment in their dads' eyes as they looked at me. I wish, as I spoke to the waitress, I could see the needs of her kids, who often had no dad at home, the eyes of kids only hoping their mom came home safe.

CHAPTER 4

I wish I had stood up for the flight attendant and told that drunk son of a bitch to sit upright and wait until after we took off for his third drink, for she was probably making $22 an hour, drove a shitty car, and was wearing heels that not only hurt her feet but were also permanently damaging her back.

I wish for a lot of things, but wishing to change what has been done is like driving backward using a rearview mirror. What I'm thankful for is that I'm becoming the man I should have been. I'm not there yet, but I'm on the right road. So, fathers, love your daughters. And if I could add, regardless of whether they are a flight attendant, a waitress, your girlfriend, or your wife, they are still someone's daughter, so treat them all like you would like your daughter to be treated.

- *As you take your daily walk, think about some of your personal regrets; all of us have them. As you look back at your life, what have you learned?*
- *Think of two special ladies in your life. Put this book down and give them a call.*

My Son

The apprehension. The excitement. The uncertainty of soon seeing a son who has been separated from me for a while, a son who is trying to be closer to me, come back into my life. Was he always there, or did he just come back? Was I receptive or elusive? What would this new chapter in our relationship hold? One of positive memories, one of regrets, one of love, or all of the above.

How horrible a dad I must have been, not knowing how great my son was at the time and judging his success against my achievements. How awful I was as a father.

One night, as he left my home in Colorado, I said goodbye at the airport—a goodbye I dreaded saying before he even came. Such a fine young man. Much more representative of his wonderful mother than me.

Oh, how I miss my son.

I've now made it a point to visit my son regularly. God gave me a second chance, and I can promise I'm not going to screw it up this time.

- *Before you go to sleep tonight, call that special man in your life. Whether it's your nephew, uncle, brother or son, tell them you love them.*
- *What was their reaction? What did you feel? When are you going to do it again?*
- *If your doctor told you your time on Earth was shortened to one year, what would you do differently?*

CHAPTER 4

To whom would you tell you love them? Why aren't you doing that now?

The Greatest Person My Kids Never Knew

In early December of 2020, I had the honor of hosting my daughter in my home for several weeks. She, like millions of other kids during COVID, was studying online and working to complete her degree. She is my somewhat emotional daughter who, when compared to her younger sister, is quiet. The truth is, anyone compared to her younger sister is quiet.

Prior to her arrival, I thought about the many activities I would like to do with her—skiing, putting up the Christmas tree, etc. I then realized that the most important thing we can do is just be present in each other's space. During her visit, I had several opportunities to observe her as she presented her MBA projects to her class via Zoom. So professional, so precise, yet with an air of humor that I lack. Clearly, she's a product of her wonderful mother.

She grew up in a military family, as I was constantly gone, never at the bus stops, and rarely involved in her school. I was climbing a ladder that I later found out was leaning against the wrong wall. Every promotion meant a new assignment, and if that meant being away from the family for a year, well, so be it, because I thought that if I reached the so-called pinnacle, then I could look back and give her and my family a better life.

Then, as expected, some of the rungs became too hard to reach, and I fell out of intimacy with my wife and my kids. Now I'm finding my internal self—a self I had forgotten, a self in need of first aid, a self that has

CHAPTER 4

changed. While climbing the wrong ladder, my absence caused irreparable damage that no amount of money could ever mend. I thank God for moving those rungs and pushing me off a ladder I didn't belong on.

People often joke with me about my likeness to the mega-great actor Denzel Washington, even nicknaming me Denzel. No different than many of you resembling Brad Pitt, Regina King, or Julia Roberts. It made for a good laugh at the time, and it still does. However, one film of Denzel's that caused me not to want to be like him was *Flight*, a fictional movie about an alcoholic pilot who sacrificed his family and, for years, focused on himself. During a routine flight, he miraculously saves an airplane from a maintenance malfunction. In the end, Denzel Washington's character admits to his alcoholism and being drunk during the flight, and as a result, he is sentenced to prison. While in prison, his estranged son, now in college, comes to visit him. They exchange hugs, and his dad says, "What's up? Tell me about school." His son looks at him and says, "Well, Dad, for school I'm writing my final paper, and I decided to write it about you. The title is the 'Greatest Person I Never Knew.'"[10]

I look at my new life now, and I ask, Did God intend that the message of that film be meant for me? No, I'm not an alcoholic, nor have I ever been arrested or sent to prison, but the message wasn't that. The message was one of not being there. I never wanted to be the greatest person my kids never knew, and it was during the time in December that my daughter stayed with

---

[10] *Flight*, Robert Zemeckis (director), 2012, Paramount, 2:18 min.

me that I became increasingly damn sure of my need to be present with my daughter and all my kids from that point on. I thank God for taking the masks of conformity and success off my face and tossing them into the trash can.

- *Who in your life would say that you are the greatest person they never knew? Why would they say that?*
- *What are you going to do to change from being the greatest person they never knew to the greatest person they know?*

Pre-Combat Checks Aren't Just For Combat

I learned the importance of pre-combat checks many years ago. Once we received our warning order, we would brief our team, assemble the necessary equipment, and then meet with our leadership for the formal operations order.

We had a similar procedure to follow once the operation order was received. As we moved forward in the planning and rehearsal of the operation, we would conduct a backbrief to ensure we understood the mission. So, if you were the third platoon leader and fifth in the order of march and had responsibility to seize Objective Bean from 270 degrees to 360 degrees to thwart a counterattack, your leadership would be expecting you to recite the major items back to your immediate leader.

The key here was to ensure you understood what you were supposed to do and for your leaders to have confidence that you understood what you were supposed to do. This event was normally non-confrontational, and initial mistakes or misunderstandings were treated with professional courtesy. Leaders who were supervising would simply tell those who did not backbrief the plan correctly, "No, that's not quite right; what I want you to do is this or that." The military held the belief that communication was not complete until those you communicated with completely understood what you said; it was never enough for the supervisor to just say it to your subordinates. The other purpose, somewhat subliminal, was to ensure that you, the subordinate, typically the execution arm, really understood the main points of the directive, so if all else failed and you lost communication, you and everyone who heard you knew the main points of what you were trying to achieve, and the mission would be successful.

If we were conducting a tactical operation by foot, once we had everything packed, we would jump up and down to verify there were no extraneous sounds. What tended to rattle was repacked. You would be surprised at what makes noise when you are trying to be quiet! It was no different than a hunter moving through the woods, trying to get that eight-point buck.

The next thing we did occurred after we left our secure perimeter but before really getting into enemy territory. We would take a knee, take our helmets off, look all around us, and just listen. The purpose of this ten- to twenty-minute pause was to get the feel of the battlefield, sense the smell, hear the environment, and just pause. This also allowed us to get a sense of what the environment should sound like as we proceeded forward.

I learned the backbrief, the jump, and the stop for silence thirty-eight years ago, and they have served me flawlessly.

Where I screwed up was when I got out of the military some fifteen years ago and put the military techniques I learned in the closet along with my uniforms. I thought the pre-combat checks were only for the military, but boy, was I wrong.

CHAPTER 4

It took me another twelve years after retiring to realize the backbrief was not to hear me say what my mission was; it was for me to understand and show my leadership and peers that I was listening. The jumping up and down wasn't about hearing or not hearing your spoon rattle against your gun; it was focused on one's personal quest to keep distractions away. The stop for silence was more than a time to adjust; it was also a time to enter another person's world.

I remember my relationship failures, and yes, they were failures. I realize that if I had just listened to my partner more, if I had respectfully said when they were done talking, "Here is what I heard you say." I know just the act of me acknowledging I heard them would have moved us leaps and bounds down the road to recovery. I was already trained to do just that, but to my demise, I never used it in my personal life.

This is a similar noise to the jumping up and down that we had to physically perform as part of our pre-combat check to see what made noise; it is a similar noise you hear on those long trips with your loved one—what a distraction, right? Well, the sound of that distraction is no different than us letting other people play roles in our personal lives.

Stopping in the woods after leaving your line of departure (your safety zone) is really focused on taking the necessary step outside of our comfort or security zone to really understand your partner's environment.

In all of my relationships, I initially ventured from what I believed was comfortable ground—my territory—into the wilderness of a new relationship. But what I did not do well, hence the failed relationships, was really stay on my knees long enough to see, understand, and sense my partner's view.

The stop to sense the environment in uniform is the same in a relationship. Both are entering new domains, and both must be given time to take the helmet off, per se, smell the environment, listen, and hopefully look at each other. Both need to just take a knee!

For those who might argue after taking a knee that some partners will split and run back to their homes, I'd say that it is also a relationship saved because those two individuals will go their separate ways and not be tied up trying to make something work that won't.

So, the next time you have an argument with a loved one or a close friend and you think the grass is greener on the other side, ask yourself if you did your pre-combat checks. Did you listen to understand, or were you just quiet? Did you shake the distractions away? Did you step into the other person's world just to say you did it, or did you really understand it? If the answer is that you could have done a better job, then there is no better time than now to reach out and tell that person what you think, and both of you can try to do a better job.

The analogy that I have used during this section was pre-combat checks, and the implied situation was how each side was preparing for a so-called enemy. What is clear and should be clear to everyone is that the pre-combat checks are checks both you and your partner need to work on to be stronger together as you face the

CHAPTER 4

world and should not be used against each other.

As I write this, I do so with a bit of sadness. The pre-combat checks I learned in the military were taught to me by our Vietnam veterans. I came into the Army during a time when the veterans of Vietnam ran our military and were still very active and involved in our training. The Vietnam veterans were leaders who perfected this practice in war, and it was these same leaders who never got the credit they deserved.

So, when our nation marvels at the Army I had the honor to serve in—an Army that beat Saddam during Desert Storm in 1991 in four days, an Army that took Grenada in three days, an Army that won every tactical engagement in Iraq and Afghanistan, an Army that achieved all those accolades and is still feared by every single adversary—know that it was trained by the Vietnam veterans of yesterday. Those are the same Vietnam veterans who came home from Vietnam to an America that spit on them, and to this day, they are in a nation that has not properly made up for the poor treatment we once gave them. How ironic! What if our nation had done its pre-combat checks to take care of the Vietnam veterans? What if our nation could have set the same example our Army did? How we as a nation could have prospered!

- *When was the last time you jumped up and down to hear what was not secure in your relationship? When was the last time you took your helmet off to really listen to a loved one?*

- *What other tools have you been taught to use, whether in business or the military, that could be applied to improve your relationships?*
- *Last point, please find a Vietnam veteran in your neighborhood and personally with your heart, thank them, not for their service but for their sacrifice. Because while others of that era were finding ways to avoid the draft, our Vietnam veterans were finding ways to serve our country!*

The PAVE Matrix

I arrived at the airport and preflighted the plane. The snow and ice were clear, and the engines were warm. It was time to start the engines and taxi to the run-up area before taking off.

After arriving at the run-up area, I performed an internal check with the engine running. My goal was to make sure that the plane would perform flawlessly in flight, so I ran the engine up to a certain RPM, typifying the power needed for flight, and I then checked the magnetos, the prop, and then the deice boots to ensure they worked. Should something arise, I would simply taxi back to the hangar and arrange to get it fixed.

As a matter of fact, when I'm doing my preflight run-up and taking off, I am purposely looking for a reason not to fly. My theory is simple: I'd rather be on the ground wishing I was in the air than be in the air wishing I was on the ground.

I think of my life and how different it would have been if I had applied the preflight principle. Had I used the same checklist before I went into the corporate world, walked into a relationship, or even started something new, how different and maybe even better things would have been.

It's not about checking to see if my hair is combed or if my shoes are shined; it's the mental part of my preflight that I tend to forget. I'm not talking about rehearsing what I'm going to say; I'm talking about asking if I'm in the right state of mind.

This, by the way, includes flying. I can't tell you how many times I've gone to the airport in ideal weather, looked at the airplane, and said, "It's just not my day." The plane was fine, but I wasn't. I can also tell you there are many days when I've gone to the airport in pouring rain with four-hundred-foot ceilings, taken off, and had a wonderful flight. So why did I successfully preflight both myself and the airplane before flying but not myself before engaging in a relationship? Well, because I was stupid!

The FAA has what's called a PAVE (**P**ilot, **A**ircraft, En**V**ironment, and **E**xternal Pressures) matrix[11] which is used as a tool for pilots to self-evaluate the conditions and themselves. It looks at the entire spectrum of the pilot (including the emotional state) and the aircraft. Every pilot goes through this checklist to see if they're ready to fly. I think it's a great checklist, but I think waiting to use it just before you are ready to fly is a bit too late. I think that checklist is something we need to use when we get out of bed and something we should use every day for activities beyond flying. Imagine how useful it would be before confronting your ex-spouse over who has the kids for Easter. Imagine how useful it would have been had you and your ex-spouse used the PAVE matrix and not had the argument that led to your separation. You could have spent Easter together with your kids in church.

---

[11] FAA PAVE Matrix, FAA.Gov, figure 2-7.

CHAPTER 4

The preflight may be noisy, cumbersome, and even a bit methodical, but it forces pilots to check their plane and themselves before launching into the wild blue yonder. I can only imagine the number of lives saved because discrepancies were found before departing and the plane and/or the pilot had a second chance to fix themselves.

As I sit lonely, divorced, without my kids, away from friends, and disconnected, I can only wonder who I would have been had I preflighted myself years ago.

- *As you move forward, try to think about how you can apply the PAVE matrix in your relationship, so you don't take off only to wish you were on the ground!*

The Great Al Jarreau

A couple of weeks ago, I got frustrated watching the mostly negative network news. What I saw about COVID, unnecessary violence, and our lost jobs made me cry. To remedy that, I did what most do: I channel-surfed.

Having already watched every James Bond movie twice or more, I settled on a TV special talking about the life of Al Jarreau. It had just begun, and given how fired up I was about the news, I knew I would be awake for a while.

For those not familiar, Al Jarreau was a jazz, blues, pop, and all-in-one singer who combined the best beats, as shown in his hits like "Rooftop" and others. But perhaps those of you fifty years old and older appreciate his more formal work like "Mornin'" or "We're in This Love Together," both former number-one hits.

The special followed the sequence of showing a song clip, then interviewing band members, then family, then an older segment showing Al. I learned some very interesting things about Al, like that he hadn't gotten a hit until he was thirty-five and that he was married for over forty years. I learned how much he loved his band members and how much they loved him. I learned how humble he was and how much he loved his son, often calling him while he was touring just to ensure he'd done his homework.

However, the one thing that stuck with me about Al

CHAPTER 4

was his desire to make a difference. I recall an interview with a bandmember named Larry who had been part of Al's band for years. During the interview, Larry recounted his final days with Al. Al's condition was terminal, and he would only accept close friends as visitors. Larry recalled that during his final visit, Al asked Larry, "Do you think we made a difference?"

Larry looked at Al and replied, "Hell yeah, Al, you changed music; not too many have that to say."

Al Jarreau passed away several days later. Al Jarreau showed it's never too late to start, to always love your family and commit to your friends, and by doing all that, he did what few others did: he made a difference in the world of music.

I often thought about the difference I've made by serving others and my country, helping raise three great kids, being a good but not great son to my parents, and frankly, not being the best companion to those I have loved. I don't know, but I wonder what I will be remembered for. Al Jarreau never had a mask. He was not impatient; he did not worry about climbing ladders, yet he changed music. What did Keith Cooper change?

- *Having visited many people who are near death, we never discussed how their stocks were doing, they never inquired about their home's value, many shared regrets, while others laid in silence and held my hand. Are you focused on making money or making a difference? No, you can't focus on both. What do you want your epitaph to say?*

Threes to Fours

As I navigated to become a better person, I decided to document my transition using the change from three words to four words.

The Threes	*The Fours*
I don't know.	I can do better.
I was wrong.	I will do better.
I am sorry.	I want your feedback.
Let's move on.	Here's what I need.
You are important.	Can you teach me?
I love you.	It's important to me.
I need help.	I disagree, let's talk.
I will improve.	
Can you help?	
I am listening.	
I respect you.	

In my many, many years of being what I thought was a good lover, a good father, a good leader, a good husband, and a good friend—all these years of not being genuine, not working on myself—at no time did I seek self-improvement, and my vocabulary was absent of the threes to the fours. Now, my vocabulary consists primarily of the threes and the fours.

But the consequences are dire.

As I sit at home, looking at the beauty of Grand County, the greatness of the landscape, the silence,

CHAPTER 4

and the peace, I'd give it all up just to say "I was wrong" to those I have wronged; "I am sorry" to those I have hurt; and "I love you" to those I have loved. I missed my opportunity. Don't miss yours. Follow the threes and take them to the fours.

- *Take a minute and put your version of threes to fours together. What are you going to do to change?*
- *Which of my threes give you the most difficulty? The most inspiration? How about the fours? Why?*

The Exit Glacier—Man, Did I Bitch

It was my daughter Megan's last day in Alaska; she would be leaving for her home in the Lower 48 after a week in Alaska. One day, we were in the beautiful port town of Seward, with mountains on one side and the spectacular Resurrection Bay on the other. Megan, unfortunately, was sick with a head cold. Her eyes were red and watery, and she looked half-asleep. My son, Chris, the "Nike" or "Let's do it" son, was feeling the opposite; he was full of energy. So after breakfast, we headed out of Seward one final time. The rain that started as a sprinkle was now resembling a Georgia rainstorm; the intensity increased, the temperature dropped to fifty-one degrees, and I thought to myself, perfect hypothermia weather.

As we departed the restaurant parking lot, I turned and asked the proverbial parent question, hoping for an answer of "No, I'm good." You know, the question you often ask just to get credit for asking the question, but you really don't want to do what you had asked? Yeah, that one. Well, I asked, "Did everyone have a good time?"

To which I was met with an astounding "yes." Feeling pretty good about myself, I asked the second question, a question I was sure both would say "no" to, a question that would be worded in such a way that only someone looking for pain would agree to.

"Is there anything else you would like to do here in Seward, in the rain, before we leave today?" The

CHAPTER 4

temperature was now fifty degrees, and the rain hit the car so hard you could hardly hear your voice.

I looked back at my sick daughter and received a resounding, "No, I'm good."

Then I turned to my son, sitting next to me, and heard, "The Exit Glacier."

I said, "What glacier?"

"The Exit Glacier," he said.

"Have you been there before?"

"Yes."

"Well, why do you want to go again?" Thinking he would laugh, he didn't. So about five miles out of Seward, I turned off the road for the Exit Glacier. After we parked in the Forest Service parking lot and stepped out of the car, we felt a harder rain than I imagined; this rain almost hurt when it hit you. My baseball cap now felt like a wet towel.

We then began our one-mile trek toward the Exit Glacier. People were coming off the path, many in the see-through one-piece ponchos that cost $3.50 at Walmart but $14.50 at the Park Ranger gift shop. They were saying how beautiful it was but cautioning us that the path did get much narrower and more slippery. I thought, wet dirt, slippery rocks, narrow? That's my kind of hike.

As we progressed along the forest service paved path that turned into a dirt path, we noticed signs of bear activity. I assured my son and daughter that with all the people walking and talking and the kids stomping in the mud puddles, the chances of even seeing a bear during this hike are about as good as hitting the jackpot in Vegas.

After the dirt trail ended, we started on this moderately steep, narrow path along wet rocks. My son, who was leaping ahead, began to slow a bit. I noticed even I was catching up with him, and I was catching up with others on the trail too. My Army infantry experience taught me where to plant my feet on wet surfaces and how to gain leverage, and soon I was the one bounding ahead in the rain with my super-duper rain jacket, which kept my body dry but transferred all the moisture to my pants. Within five minutes, my feet, underwear, hands, and pants were soaked. As we approached the glacier, there was a low bank of clouds; it was a bit hazy but beautiful. We snapped some pictures, and the smile on my kids' faces made the extra trip to the Exit Glacier worth it.

As we headed back down the trail toward the car, it was slippery. I found myself extending my hand to people I didn't know, helping them up the hills we were walking down. One young lady with a baby on her back reached out to me for help. I thought, Man, she must trust me. All of those I assisted by extending a hand kindly expressed what a gentleman I was for helping them, thanking me with sincerity.

After a group of people passed, I brought my two kids together on top of the slippery rock and told them how important it was to experience life while you still could. Take time with your kids when they are young to

CHAPTER 4

explore, regardless of the weather. Having all the money in the world, only to wait until you are physically challenged to use it, is not the way to enjoy life. Tie yourself to those you love, not your job. I said to the kids, I treasure my time off now, and I don't know if I'll ever go back to working in an office.

We continued down the trail toward the car, both kids smiling. Even Megan was feeling better. As we got in the car, I knew God had me turning off and following my son's desire for a reason. I knew this was the lesson I was to learn and pass on to my kids today.

As we drove from the Exit Glacier and merged onto Highway 1, we soon arrived at the Portage Flats, an open swampy area of wind coming down Turnagain Arm toward Portage Pass. The trees swayed sideways while rain pounded the car. I turned and asked with a smirk, "Does anyone want to go anywhere else before we arrive in Anchorage?"

Chris replied, "To Whittier."

To Whittier we went, and this time I didn't bitch.

- *Close your eyes and think of a time you went off the beaten path to a place you really didn't want to go. Maybe it was a wrong turn, maybe it was a different way home. Did that change open your eyes a bit? It took the Exit Glacier at fifty-one degrees to make me understand, listen, and share a life lesson with my kids. What is it going to take for you to share an important lesson with yours?*
- *Where is your Exit Glacier?*

Faith: It's Off Or On–There's No In-Between

I no longer work. I lost my lover. I lost my mom to cancer. I almost lost my house due to a forest fire. I had COVID. WTF? Why can't God let me use the dimmer switch? Why is my life made up of "off" and "on," with no subtle changes?

Could I have tried to keep the ones I love? My mom declined surgery that may have prolonged her life. Why? By the way, who the hell caused the forest fire that came within three miles of my home, the second largest fire in Colorado history? And who had the nerve to give me COVID? God, where is the dimmer switch?

I barely comprehended the most recent month of my life, or rather, the last two years. But I do know a lot happened all at once—a lot that I and others were unprepared for. COVID hit everyone like a train, and with all other things going on in my personal life, well, it was like being tied to the train tracks. Where is the sympathy, the care? Was I just not ready for this catastrophe?

Was this a warning of what could come? Our nation was a mess, and so was I. What should I do? What difference can I really make? Why do so many bad things happen to me and, I'm sure, others, all at once? Can't there be a progression of bad and a suddenness of good? I mean, isn't there a way to focus our lives so only good things happen at once? But bad things—well,

CHAPTER 4

bad things need to be incremental so we can handle them, right?

Each night before going to sleep, I used to use the dimmer, slowly watching the lights go down to almost a flicker. Now, I flip the switch off. I accept that my life no longer has a dimmer switch; you make your own luck. I clearly now understand the importance of being "on" or "off," with no in-between. I realized after that one simple act of the dimmer switch that God was trying to teach me that my faith is either "off" or "on," no in-between, no gradual acceptance. Because in the process of all the issues occurring to me, I was losing faith.

Thank you, God, for taking away my thoughts of a dimmer switch and allowing me to commit fully to You.

- *Have you ever tried to give God advice? How did that go for you?*
- *What is going on in your life to cause turmoil? Perhaps you should consider changing the narrative from "Why me, God?" to "God, what are you trying to teach me?"*

My Date With Sadie

I arrived early to pick her up. It was a cool Georgia evening in 1981, and we had planned to go to a nice dinner and a movie. I wore a collared shirt and a sweater to keep the cold out. When I arrived, I knocked on the door and heard a distant voice say, "Come on in, I'm getting ready." I had some flowers I purchased at the base flower shop earlier in the day, and although they looked a bit wilted, they were still pretty. I placed them on the living room table. As I sat down and looked around, I saw a neat home, maybe even too neat—everything was in place and impressive. I thought, is this the way she always is, or is it just a first impression for me? I could hear movement in the back, obviously her getting dressed, and combined with the "I'll be right out," it was quite entertaining.

As I looked around, I saw a door open just a crack. Something said look, so when I glanced over, I saw the most beautiful big brown eyes I'd guess were about three feet above the floor, clearly a youngster. Once we made eye contact, there was a slam, followed by a sound saying, "What did I tell you? We are not going out until they leave." I thought, Who are "they?" Maybe me? Who was the owner of those beautiful eyes?

Now I was curious, so I kept looking in that direction, knowing the door would soon open again. So, I got up from the couch and moved near the door, and when it opened, I said, "Hi."

Those eyes stared at me and replied, "Hello."

CHAPTER 4

It was a young child in a room with the babysitter. The babysitter quickly came to apologize and said how sorry she was when the little girl came out of her room.

I replied, "No reason to apologize."

After the introductions, I now knew that my date had a little daughter, Sadie, a special daughter who had Down syndrome. As I squatted down in the room next to her, I picked up her toys and started playing with them. She quickly sat right next to me, letting me know the names of her dolls while we both tried to squeeze into this little Barbie house in the corner. I didn't fit. As I played with Sadie, I wondered why my date didn't mention she had a child, not to mention a special child. I rationalized that it was our first real date, and she didn't want to tell me, but why put a child in a separate room?

Yes, my date was my age, twenty-one, and Sadie was probably six, meaning a teenage pregnancy. It seemed like the two minutes we played together were fifteen minutes. Soon, the babysitter started in our conversation, and I learned about the girl who is now dating the guy she liked, her favorite and worst teachers, and even the latest dance—The Dog (don't ask, remember it's 1981 in Columbus, Georgia).

Sadie began to serve us all tea (make-believe, of course) when my date, looking like a million bucks, came out of her room and walked in on us. She was seemingly surprised to see me hunched over, sipping tea next to a Barbie playhouse with her daughter, laughing, and the babysitter going on with her teenage drama, talking away.

She politely asked me to come into the living room. We sat down, and she took my hand and explained that she got pregnant at a young age and decided to keep the baby. Every guy she'd dated in the past few years since the baby's father left was turned off by knowing about her child's disability, not to mention that she had a child out of wedlock. It was not something she planned to hide forever from anyone; she just wanted to wait until the right time. I looked down, looked up, and said, "I'm sorry."

She quickly replied, "Don't be. Down syndrome is common; there are numerous therapies invented every day. I'm learning to be a nurse, and I'm on top of the latest technology."

I then interrupted what seemed to be a planned speech by her and said, "I know she'll be okay. You're the one I'm worried about." I then proceeded to tell her that anyone who would hide someone as beautiful as Sadie or any member of their family for any reason needed help. If the other guys she dated felt differently, then maybe they were the wrong guys for her. Around that time, Sadie came running out into the living room to let me know my tea was getting cold. Her mom replied, "Keith and I are leaving." Sadie's jubilant face turned sad, and that change of expression made me say, "No, no, we're not leaving; how about pizza?"

In 1981, we did not have delivery, so we got on her rotary phone and dialed the local pizza place. I jumped into my car to go get it. I came back and put it on the

CHAPTER 4

living room floor, where the babysitter, my date, Sadie, her dolls, and I sat and ate our dinner.

As we finished chatting, my date turned the TV to a show and sat next to me; Sadie was on one side, my date on the other, and the babysitter was continuing her tirade about school and boys. We weren't paying any attention.

After a while, I felt a weight on my shoulder. Sadie's head now rested on me, and she was sound asleep. My date asked the babysitter to call her mom to be picked up, and she said she would pay her for the entire evening, to which the babysitter said, "Right on!" (that was what cool people said back then).

Once the babysitter's mom arrived, my date got up, paid the babysitter, thanked her, and then put Sadie to bed. She came back, sat across, and looked at me. I could see the appreciation and compassion in her eyes; I could also see the sadness for what she had done. She said, "This was the best date I've ever had; when can I see you again?" I looked at her for what seemed to be ten minutes but was only a few seconds, then replied, "The evening was fine, but you won't see me again." I asked her to take time to work on herself from the inside and to give me a call in a few years if she was still interested.

It's been forty years. I've had no calls, but I know she's working on herself and is a better person.

I now look back and wish I had taken the advice I gave her. I wish I had been the man my dad was in January 1961 when he married my mom, a Black woman with an eight-year-old daughter and a one-year-old son, and given her and Sadie another chance with me.

I should have stayed and dated Sadie's mom, for in the end, it was me who ran from reality, not her. God taught me that important lesson in 1981: that I was starting to wear the mask of conformity and trying to teach someone I didn't know well before I taught myself.

- *Take a second und think: Have you ever wished you had taken the medicine you prescribed to someone else?*
- *Who are you teaching before you are taught?*

The I-Should-Haves

I woke up one morning at 4:34 a.m. The bright moonlight made it look like the sun was out as it reflected off the snow. The sun, however, was still sleeping, and I had three hours of shut-eye before it would bless us with its radiance. The moon was doing a pretty good imitation for those who were awake.

Why did I wake up? What was on my mind? Well, it wasn't the moonlight, that's for sure. I had a case of the "I-should-haves." You know, "I should've done the dishes last night," or "I should've gone to the store before they ran out of the crackers I enjoy," or the best one, "I should've finished the email I was working on before going to bed."

Well, all those are true, but really, I should've woken up for the wonderful women in my life.

I should've thanked my ex-wife during Christmas and told her how great she was for raising our wonderful kids.

I should've told my daughter I loved her last night before hanging up the phone.

I should've told my ex-girlfriend, Yes, we will buy that home on the lake, any lake, if it would help to keep you in my life.

I should've addressed the checkout clerk by her name and thanked her for helping me at the supermarket yesterday afternoon.

I should've walked into the coffee shop, bought a $20 gift card, and given it to a teacher.

I should've walked more and held more hands.

God woke me up to let me know that "I should have" doesn't involve chores or work. It involves love and respect.

- *What are your "I-should-haves"?*
- *What did you not do that you should have done? What are you going to do about it?*
- *Turn and look into your partner's eyes. Name two cashiers at the grocery store you shop at each week. If you don't shop, then tell each other the first name of the parking attendant at the lot or garage you park at each weekday. Make a commitment to each other to thank them the next time you see them.*

What Counts Is Getting Back Up

My sister, Beatrice, was about eight years older than me. In the late sixties and early seventies, the only time I have accurate memories of us being in the same household, I remember she listened to the coolest music like "Killing Me Softly" sung by Roberta Flack, "Rescue Me" by Freda Payne, and "Up, Up, and Away" by the 5th Dimension. I recall putting my ear to her door just to hear the cool music and dancing, or what I call popping my fingers and trying to dance. Yes, I tended to eavesdrop on her as she danced. One song I vividly remember was sung by The Stylistics. It was called "Break Up to Make Up."

Remember, music reflects our time. The sixties and seventies were periods of change in America. Perhaps nothing is more reflective of documenting that change than the singer-songwriter Marvin Gaye's 1972 album, *What's Going On*.

Back to the seventies and The Stylistics: why do we break up to make up? Well, in truth, after fifty years have passed, I'm convinced The Stylistics had a deeper message. It wasn't solely the breakup as much as it was the makeup; it was the feeling of the makeup that caused the breakup. No one goes to a boxing match in hopes of a first-round knockout; we go to see twelve to fifteen rounds of knockout, drag-out fighting. Fighting that ultimately might cause one opponent to fall down, giving him an opportunity to define his greatness when he stands up again. Imagine if Rocky never got up after

Apollo Creed knocked him down the first time. It would've been the end of the series without a statue in Philadelphia, not to mention a *Rocky V*.

So, as I go through life consistently getting knocked down and seeing others get knocked down, I no longer judge the knockdown, which could be otherwise known as the break-up. I judge how and if they, and I, get back up. The make-up.

At one time or another, all of us feel this anxiety, this fear, and we transmit what's happened to us. All of us go through this sense that things are not going to get better. We must understand that by changing nothing, nothing changes.

So, I ask you, next time you get knocked down, what are you going to change? Because if you are like me, getting knocked down is almost a routine now, and God made it clear: it's all about how I get up.

- *Have you ever broken up in a relationship just to feel the awesome power of making up? If so, then why don't you apply that same thought to how you can rise above your current problems and get back on your feet?*
- *God knows you are going to make mistakes. Reach out your hand the next time you are down and let Him help you up; make up with Him.*

Why I Do It

It's the bald head of the kids who should have hair.

It's the scrawniness of the adults who should be muscular.

It's the pain on the forehead of those parents and loved ones who are worried.

It's for the dogs who no longer have the kids to pull their tails or sleep on their stomachs.

It's for the dads so they can have tea parties with their five-year-olds inside the Barbie house.

It's for the moms who still need time to show their daughters how to apply makeup.

It's for the parents to be able to interrogate their kid's date before the prom.

It's so sons and daughters can bury their moms and dads, not the other way around.

It's so we give medical technology time to progress and maybe find a cure.

It's so death becomes natural.

It's to allow kids time to take their first communion or bar mitzvah.

It's so the young adults who are summer camp counselors can meet, fall in love, and raise a family.

I do it because I care.

I do it because I'm human.

I do it because I'm a child of God.

I wrote this story to address the questions of those who ask me why I volunteer. The many who seem confused as to how I can find time. Well, having lost both my parents and my sister to cancer, I realize that my purpose means more than my comfort.

- *Should giving back be extra or an exception? Part of John 14:12 says "...the works that I do he will do also; and greater words than these he will do..." What are you doing to give back?*

Four Bags Of Concrete

There are two days until Christmas, and I'm sitting on four bags of Quikrete concrete and couldn't be happier. Let me tell you just how I got here.

It started with a tornado—yes, a tornado that ripped its way through several states. I could no longer just sit or just write a check; I had to act. So, I decided to stop watching TV and start moving. On Wednesday, ten days before Christmas 2021, I received the note I was expecting regarding how I could help the tornado victims in Western Kentucky. I went and bought a lot of diapers, toys, and bedding, loaded those items into my plane, and flew them to Western Kentucky, specifically Mayfield. At the same time, I contacted and received confirmation that my St. Bernard Project (SBP) volunteer request had been approved for New Orleans or Houston. I chose New Orleans.

So, after dropping off supplies, on Sunday, the nineteenth, I departed Kentucky, landing at the Lakefront Airport in New Orleans at about 4:00 p.m.

The next three days were filled with volunteering to support a project to rebuild a home for a family in need, a home destroyed during Hurricane Ida.

The first day I learned how to install flooring; the second day I dug holes for a cistern; and on my last day we were putting down the concrete, hence why I was sitting on four bags of concrete during lunch.

I was so impressed by the young kids, all volunteers

with the St. Bernard Project or AmeriCorps. There's Cleo from New Orleans; he's my supervisor, all of twenty-five years old. Then there's Peter; he brings our supplies. And Max. Max is the St. Bernard Project philosopher; he finds humor and fault in everything we're trying to do. And then there's Herb, the improviser. Together, we make up a team of volunteers who, although very different on the outside, are absolutely the same inside.

Everyone seems intrigued by my presence. I'm easily twice their age, but I never told them how old I was. When they asked where I was from, I said Colorado, not Winter Park. I never said I flew my own plane to New Orleans, parked just two miles away at the general aviation airport, nor would I bring up my other volunteer references over the past nine years straight, minus COVID. I just said that I was off work and how proud I was to be here.

At lunch, I didn't have any food; I wasn't hungry because documenting this special time was more important. The family that will occupy this home—a young boy, his mom and his grandmother—just departed. The mom and grandmother were talking to our supervisor about the progress and then discussing among themselves what furniture goes where while their young boy staked out his claim to the yard as he set up his baseball diamond made of rocks.

Their happiness and the young boy's joy brought tears to my eyes. Soon those of us working would be done with our break, and I'd have four more hours to

CHAPTER 4

volunteer until we were all finished. I wished I could stay, but they were closing shop until the twenty-seventh to allow everyone time to go home for the holidays.

I've been in a lot of places and worn some nice clothes, but, except for my time at the cabin, I've never been as happy as when I'm volunteering. And for that hour, my happy place was sitting on four bags of concrete. I hoped my time in New Orleans had made a small difference in someone's life just forty-eight hours before Christmas. God had placed me where I belonged.

- *How did you feel the last time you volunteered your time? Wouldn't you agree the only gift you will ever want again in life is the gift to take the time off to do it again?*

- *Now think as you look out your window. When are you planning on holding down four bags of concrete?*

Whose Name Would I Call?

As I lay on the bed, eight days before Christmas in New Orleans, I picked up the remote and started channel surfing, not really paying attention but looking at each channel the same. Suddenly, I saw an ad with two of my favorite singers, Carole King and James Taylor. I've seen both in concert and love their music, not to mention their songwriting ability. So I listened and watched. It was an upcoming CNN special with the two discussing their careers, their friendship, and their lives. It was titled "You've Got a Friend." I thought, How cute! That's the name of the song they once sang together. I then watched a little bit more as the announcer advertised the special, all the while hearing the background singing of the song with the lyrics "Just call out my name." I learned when the special would be aired, then turned off the TV and ventured out to grab a bite to eat on Bourbon Street.

I walked along the not-so-busy street, given that it was raining and the temperature was forty-nine degrees, awfully cold for Louisiana. And as I walked, I thought about the upcoming special while humming "You've Got a Friend" and asked myself, who would I call? I walked by numerous restaurants, looking through the glass at people together, and thought, well, they have someone to call, but what about me? Who would I call? I went to a bar and sat on a barstool next to some couples and people by themselves, all watching the Saints-Buccaneers game, and as I ate the double

CHAPTER 4

cheeseburger with onion rings, I listened to the Creole chant of words about the Buccaneers I could not understand. I thought, who would I call?

During the short two-block walk to the hotel, the restaurants, bars, and strip clubs I passed didn't catch my attention, but the thought of "who would I call?" did keep my attention. My parents are in heaven with my sister. I lost my love, who I would normally call, and like most relationships, when you lose the one you love, you lose the family and friends who are attached to the one you loved. I don't have a lot of true friends. So, who would I call? I finally realized that I don't need to worry about calling anyone's name because I don't have to. I now know that when I need a friend, I will call God's name. Not as a last resort but as the first choice.

- *Take a deep breath. How many times have you called out someone's name for help and not received it? Personally, I've fallen into the trap of calling and either not getting a response or being told they can help me after they complete the sixteen items ahead of my request.*

- *COVID caused me to be more appreciative of my friends, to not take them for granted, and to forgive. Now with my dad, mom, and sisters in heaven and only a few real close friends, I rely on God. Who do you rely on?*

About The Author

Keith Cooper is a native of Anchorage, Alaska. After graduating from West Point, he served in the Army Infantry for 26 years where he commanded from platoon to brigade level receiving the Distinguished Service Medal, Bronze Star, and three-time recipient of the Legion of Merit. Following Keith's military career, he went to work in the aerospace and defense sectors, working for three large defense companies before starting his own company, One Core Consultants. Keith's interests revolve around learning, traveling, hiking, volunteering, and writing. He has flown over eighty-five missions in support of those needing cancer treatment. He is also an animal lover and has personally flown over a hundred animals from shelters to foster and permanent homes. He recently completed the Camino Frances pilgrimage, a 500 mile walk from France across the Pyrenees to Santiago, Spain. He is the father of three wonderful kids and splits his time between Alaska and Colorado.

Printed in the USA
CPSIA information can be obtained
at www.ICGtesting.com
LVHW041207070224
770827LV00007B/37